M000084533

Defeat Cancer
A Battle Plan for Living

How I Fought Cancer
and live Cancer Free Today!

NOTE FROM THE PUBLISHER

Defeat Cancer represents the experience and views of the author and not the publisher. Claims for healing through the use of the natural treatments described in *Defeat Cancer* are the belief of the author and not the publisher. While KiwE Publishing believes that a healthy lifestyle is a great preventative and restorative, the success of the author in defeating cancer in the long term (full remission) remains to be determined. The reader is encouraged to use good judgment in the treatment of any cancer, consult with and consider the full spectrum of medical and natural options.

Neil D. Holland, publisher
KiwE Publishing, Ltd.

Defeat Cancer
A Battle Plan for Living

How I Fought Cancer
and live Cancer Free Today!

by
Gregory A. Gore

PUBLISHING

Copyright: Gregory A. Gore, 2006

All rights reserved. No part of this publication may be reproduced, stored in a retrieval system, or transmitted in any form or by any means — electronic, mechanical, photocopy, copy, recording, or any other — except for brief quotations in printed reviews, without the prior written permission of the publisher.

Published:
KiwE Publishing, Ltd.
Spokane, Washington
http://www.kiwepublishing.com

Library of Congress Control Number: 2006934229
ISBN   10 1-933973-02-1
          13 978-1-933973-02-9

Cover Photo by Matthew Gore, Lucid Lens Productions; Anchorage, Alaska

EXCULPATORY NOTE

Let it be known that the author, publisher, and/or companies and brand names mentioned, will not be held liable for injury or damage allegedly arising from the use of information and/or products mentioned in this book.

In this book I talk about products I have used to win my battle with cancer. My only intent is to explain what all the items mentioned in this book did for me, and/or what I have learned about them and allow you to decide for yourself whether any of this information may be beneficial to you.

Let me emphasize! I do not claim any of the nutrients, products, or supplements listed within this book will cure you of cancer or any other disease, nor do the companies of the products I use, or have mentioned, make any such claim.

I only mention the products in each category I personally used to stop my cancer. In no way am I paid for mentioning any of the products I have used or still use. Nor do I wish to appear to endorse them. There are other products available that also contain the same or similar nutrients as the products I mention. These products and the information in this book are, however, the ones I found that worked best for me to fight my cancer and drastically lowered my Prostate-Specific Antigen (PSA) levels.

If you choose to use any of the products mentioned within this book, with or without your doctor's consent, you and only you are responsible, and you do so at your own risk.

You should always check with your doctor or licensed medical practitioner about decisions regarding what products you might start taking, need to be taking, or are thinking about changing or stopping.

This book and its reference pages are in no way intended as a substitute for the diagnoses, treatment, and/or advice of a qualified licensed professional.

At no time in this book do I intend or attempt to sway your opinion one way or another; give medical advice; treat, cure, or prevent any disease, regardless of how I may have worded my explanations.

The statements you will read in this book, other than direct quotes of others, are solely my opinion, views, or statements of what I have learned about products and procedures, and what I believe these products have done for me personally.

This book is strictly for informational and educational purposes.

Gregory A. Gore, author *Defeat Cancer*

Printed in the United States of America

Table of Contents

Dedication

I dedicate this book to my wife, who has stood by my side throughout this ordeal, her determination to help when we initially found out I had cancer and through the time when my cancer returned more aggressively to take my life. Her love and support will always be greatly appreciated. And my son, Westley Gore, for being "the key" to the early detection of my cancer.

I also dedicate this book to the memory of my father, who was diagnosed with Amyotrophic Lateral Sclerosis (ALS) in his 50s. I have never seen someone fight so hard for life and endure such pain and suffering, all the while learning about nutritional products from my mother, which helped him fight his disease and live a longer life. He will always be remembered and admired.

And I dedicate this book to the many doctors who have risked their licenses and livelihoods to expose the real truth about why our cancer industry is still in the dark ages on finding a cure for cancer and other degenerative diseases when it is so clear the answer is staring us in the face. This is a big reason why more and more people are turning to alternative options as a way of life to solve their health problems.

Lastly, I want to acknowledge the people who have lost their lives to cancer, thinking their only option was to follow the advice given to them by the medical community.

Note From The Author

Every effort has been made to ensure the information contained in this book is accurate. I kept it short, easy to read, and understand. The content reflects my views and the result of scientific and other research studies that I found. The reference pages comprise a wealth of information to read and study.

This book is a testimonial and story of what happened to me during my fight to overcome cancer and was written specifically to educate and inform.

For a listing of my personal websites please see page 209.

A Special Thank You

A special thank you to my mother, Louise Gore, who is an international-award-winning writer and poet. Her inspiration and continued support will always be remembered.

Also, special thanks to Rick Vassar for his interest and willingness to help with his knowledge of editing.

Preparing for Battle

If you're taking the time to read this book, you may be one of the many people who have developed some type of life-altering illness or disease. Battling this illness may be the biggest challenge of your life and may consume your every thought. If you have found out that *you* have a life-threatening disease, join the other million or more currently battling the same kind of problem that you may have, right now! Take a minute and think what you have learned about your disease on your own since you found out.

Are you starting to pull away from family and friends, people who care about you, and sincerely want to help? One of those people you shut out could be that one person who cares the most. Don't push them away. Not too long ago, this was somewhat of a problem for me. We all just want the problem to go away. Find your inner strength to let them help you in your time of need. This kind of problem is too big to fight by yourself. Face the problem head-on and prepare to win.

Be strong and move forward. Listen to what others have to say, especially the ones that have been through this ordeal and *have* done something about it as I have. I had cancer and I fought it hard, and learned a great deal along the way. Do something to keep your mind active and think positive thoughts.

Read and educate yourself on your disease and stay involved in the process. It's extremely important to have a plan of action with your medical and/or alternative therapy doctor. Think about how you're going to win this battle and follow through with the plan you have prepared. If you're angry, look within, but also look what our culture has created in our diet and lifestyle for consumers. Whatever you do, don't take it out on others. Believe it or not, anger and/or a negative attitude can, and has been proven to, actually cause and significantly contribute to poor health and disease.

Think positive thoughts and keep an open mind through this hard time. It greatly helps with the healing process. Be respectful and kind and the world will open up for you and you will see things differently. Remember, you are fighting for your life and you are not the only one with a serious problem. Take advantage of the information in this book and you will stand to benefit from it and see your rewards. But don't stop here. Keep right on going. You will reach the point where you can say, "My disease doesn't scare me anymore," and you will start to heal.

Believe in your creator and pray. Believe in yourself and laugh, love, and cry. Get in touch with your body, your spirit, your feelings, and your life. If you blame yourself, forgive yourself, and move forward to win your battle.

It is a proven fact that when we are happy it starts a flow of endorphins in our bodies that can help strengthen the immune system. This will help in the process to fight, slow or rid our bodies of disease.

Starting over to fight your disease and become healthier is hard to do when you have done things the same way your whole life. Look at it as a challenge and challenge yourself. Get out of or avoid very stressful situations and start over if needed. Take a deep breath and slow down. Take the time to walk with a loved one, breathe the air and smell the roses. This alone will start the healing process. Don't wait, get started now. Reach out to that person or people who want to help you. Your life depends on it. And yes, *you* are a special person. Believe it.

Preface

This book was started from notes I compiled in desperation to try and save my life from prostate cancer. Through my research, I discovered many of the products I mention drastically helped rebuild my immune system and helped my body kill cancer cells. I also found that many other diseases are greatly helped or corrected when you eat the correct food for your specific blood type (A,B,AB, or O). Not everybody can eat the same food and benefit from it the same way.

We desperately need to boost our immune systems so our bodies can start to heal themselves. The question is, should we try to rebuild our immune system by taking prescription drugs or should we rebuild it with superior nutritional products that our bodies desperately need and prefer? Remember this! With the many kinds of processed foods we eat today, *our bodies are screaming for nutrients.* Think about that. This is only the beginning of the problems we have today. Nutrition or prescription, it's up to you.

From my years of study I found that most cancers are symptoms of an ineffective immune system from a toxic overload of poisonous chemicals, heavy metals, processed foods, a lack of water, oxygen deprivation, and a pH imbalance, which encourage disease.

Now, I know it *is* possible to chase cancer away and slow or stop disease in order to live a better life. It is easy to get started on a good nutritional program but not as easy to stay on one, unless you're dedicated to the cause.

If you're currently struggling with cancer or another disease, I ask you not to give up but start changing your life for the better and get started on the road to recovery. Educate yourself and find out about the wonders of nutrition that are put here for all of us to use to live a healthier life. As you read this book, you will see you're not alone in this fight. Don't give up on your search. You will find a lot of the information you need right here.

Our bodies desperately need the correct amount of water, and we need to detoxify and cleanse our bodies of heavy metals, toxic chemicals, and parasites. We each need the correct diet plan, essential whole-food nutritional supplements and herbs, the proper amount of oxygen, and the correct pH balance in our bodies. We also need to exercise and get plenty of sunshine to stay healthy. I believe all these things working together is the secret to long-term health.

Introduction

Do you have cancer or another life-threatening disease? Are you ready to be healthier and have more energy? The time has come to take a long hard look at what might be happening inside your body right now.

This book outlines my search to find answers and products for fighting cancer and other diseases, and why cancer has not been eradicated over the years, especially after President Nixon declared "war on cancer" in 1971. I talk mostly about different kinds of nutritional products and cancer-fighting foods, herbs, diet, and a "Ten-Step Natural Health Plan" I have used to rid myself of this terrible disease. I also went off all medication given to me by my urologist, including radiation treatments I would have started had I stayed with his suggested treatments.

One million people or more will be diagnosed with cancer and over 500,000 others will die of this dreadful disease in the United States, in 2006. One thing you shouldn't do is sit by and wonder if it's going to be you, or a family member, who receives a diagnosis of cancer during this period. What you should do is become more involved in your health, enough to start finding out how to avoid this terrible disease.

Our medical society claims to be looking for a "cure" for cancer, something that would target and kill cancer cells. I have learned chemotherapy does not target only cancer cells. It adversely affects all our cells, and kills far more normal cells than cancer cells. Chemotherapy also damages cells that survive the treatments, leaving a cancer patient extremely weak with a badly damaged immune system. This leaves the body extremely vulnerable to other germs. I have found natural products, like whole food supplements, herbs and a super cancer diet I still follow today. All this really helped to fight my cancer and these same products can also help with other diseases.

There are nutritional products on the market today that will help the body kill cancer cells, not harm the good cells, and maintain a healthy, properly functioning immune system. The products I mention in this book are products I still use today.

If only a small amount of the money spent on cancer research each year was spent studying alternative medicine, cancer would probably not be around tomorrow. Some medical doctors in this field are saying,

"Cancer research is in the 'dark ages' and is being held back by government agencies so a real cure can't be found. They are only interested in the profitable treatments of the symptoms of the disease." Is this the real truth?

I do believe most doctors care about their patients, but they are held back by the same controlling government agencies. Check out these books to start with:

1. *Cancer Cover-Up: The Neal Deoul Story*, by Neal Deoul.
2. *Alive and Well*, by Dr. Binzel, M.D.
3. *Politics in Healing: The Suppression and Manipulation of American Medicine*, by Daniel Haley.

Doctor Binzel, and two of these authors above, put their license and/or livelihood on the line to show the real truth as many others have, and these are just a few of many other books that talk about this subject. Also, go to: *www.mercola.com/article/cancer/cancer_options.htm*.

Several natural ways have been found to fight cancer. Some are excellent and some are not so good. I believe the only thing today that will prevent the spread of cancer is our body's own defenses. This means we must have a strong immune system and keep it working at its best. The correct foods (live foods) and nutritional supplements will build our immune systems so our bodies can fight disease and continue operating at optimum efficiency. Eating the wrong foods (dead foods) will not do this for us and our bodies will pay the price of poor nutrition with disease eventually setting in.

From my research, I have found that "orthodox" (Western) medicine treats only the symptoms of cancer, not the cause. But, "alternative" medicine tells us the tumor being treated is a symptom of the cancer, and the cancer is a symptom of a weakened immune system. Alternative medicine is not concerned with the symptoms, but directly treats the cause of the disease. Read that again so it makes sense. Alternative medicine also says "cancer can be cured by fundamentally changing the bodies chemistry that created the cancer," so we should support the immune system by supplying our bodies with life-giving nutrients, herbs and special diets. We must also flush our bodies of chemical buildup (detoxify), kill parasites in our bodies (parasite cleanse), build our immune systems (immune support), and oxygenate, alkalize, and supplement our bodies with good foods, herbs, and nutritional products, so our bodies and immune systems stay healthy. Most importantly, we must give our bodies plenty of pure, fresh water every day, exercise, and learn to breathe deeply and expand our lungs, to increase our oxygen intake.

It is extremely important that we learn about the correct foods that keep our bodies alkaline instead of acidic for a strong immune system, and the correct foods for our particular blood type and metabolic type. Changing to a selective vegetarian diet when a disease is present, or before, can help to clean and detoxify our system. This was a total change of lifestyle from where I was six years ago and was definitely a change for the better.

I encourage everyone to change their lives for the better by eating correctly, supplementing their bodies with the right nutrients and learning how to maintain a "change in lifestyle," not only for their health and happiness, but for their families and, believe it or not, for generations to come. Let me clarify this a little better! If you're planning a family and you're eating foods with toxic chemicals and heavy metals, these toxins may alter your DNA. In turn, you may pass your altered DNA on to your children and grandchildren and very likely pass these abnormalities down the family tree. If this happens, your offspring will not have the opportunity to reverse these problems. Remember that more and more foods have chemicals sprayed on them, and injected into them, than ever before. This is another excellent reason to start living a healthier life. Go to: *www.curezone.com/clark* and *www.naturalhealthschool.com/acid-alkaline.html.*

In today's world, our bodies are screaming for the proper nutrients to help guard us against disease. Even the best foods today do not have the same amount of nutrients as they did 20 to 50 years ago. Our fruits and vegetables are partially depleted of very important nutrients, grown in polluted soils, sprayed with chemicals, and watered with more chemicals, and many are now genetically modified.

Life can be wonderful when we have our health. A lot of us take the benefits of a healthy life for granted, abusing our bodies with drugs, alcohol, tobacco, foods containing preservatives, artificial sweeteners, and other chemicals in and on our foods and not taking proper precautions when using or being around toxic chemicals, until it's too late. Then what do we do? We start to medicate ourselves with over-the-counter medications for headaches and aches and pains. As our health problems get worse we start to wonder what's going on, not looking at the big picture, but looking for a quick fix. We start to medicate even more with prescription medication until our doctor eventually gives us a name for the disease we may now have. We start taking more medication for the problems we now have and sometimes to counteract the problems or side effects from the medication we are already taking. As time goes on, if our disease is cancer, it's time to operate, burn it with radiation, poison our bodies with chemotherapy drugs, and possibly inject us with radioactive seeds, for certain types of cancers. If these toxic medications don't put the cancer into remission, we are sent home to die, with some wondering if they made the right decision.

This is the road I was on and I decided it was not the road I wanted to follow. So I made a U-turn and ran the other way. I made my decision to go with nutritional products, herbs, a cancer diet, and ten specific ways to stay healthy that I list later in this book, and I have not turned back since. Now that I have chased my cancer away I have proven to myself what I did, and continue to do, is really working. It was the right way for *me* to go.

This book started out of desperation and determination, from my need to learn the real truth about what I really needed to be putting in my mouth and the supplements I needed to be taking, to stop my cancer. I also talk a little on the political aspect of this subject. When you really start digging through all the information available out there, it's hard to ignore the truth.

Remember, as you read this book, I am not a doctor, but then, most medical doctors' training includes very little information on nutrition or nutritional products by the time they graduate from medical school. Now, in recent months, I see more medical schools with classes in nutrition.

I have studied and researched hundreds of scientific research papers, websites, books and pamphlets over the last six years, and started writing pertinent information down to remind myself of what I needed to be doing. Now, as this book has grown, I have tried to make it easy to read and understand so you can have a better idea about nutritional products. If you're eating what some call the "typical American diet" of refined foods (cakes, cookies, pastries, sugars, artificial sweeteners) or fast foods, deep-fried foods with transfatty acids (French fries, potato chips etc.), you are heading down the wrong road to a very unhealthy lifestyle, which can lead to disease if not corrected. These foods are acid-forming and contain life-threatening toxins. This in turn lets viruses, bacteria, mold, yeast, and fungus run wild and thrive in our bodies.

We desperately need good organic vegetables and fruits, vitamins, minerals, protein, enzymes, and more to stay healthy. I have found several foods, diets, supplements, and herbs to help fight disease and kill cancer cells, which I mention in this book. Also, if you smoke, drink in excess, or use illegal drugs, prescription drugs or over-the-counter drugs excessively, it can compound the problem you will encounter and will not give your body the fighting chance it needs to heal itself. *Prevention* is the key word, and it is affordable. You will see this word, a few more times, throughout this book.

I am one person out of many who has taken this matter very seriously, because my life depends on it. You too, must learn how to keep yourselves healthy and disease free for a better and healthier life. Before getting into this book any further, settle in with your favorite herbal tea for some really great information. We'll talk about coffee later.

PART 1

———

LET'S START WITH ME

ABOUT THE AUTHOR

Throughout my life, I have seen quite a few close friends develop some type of disease. Most developed some type of cancer and a few were terminal. But, as cancer had not touched my life up to this time I kept thinking, like most of us, it would never happen to me. And why would it? I was exercising when I had time and I was eating correctly, most of the time. However, in 1998 I started having prostate problems and was put on antibiotics by my urologist for a possible infection. After a year, and a few more appointments, we decided to do a biopsy for cancer. Within a week the results came back positive and prostate cancer was diagnosed. It was the day after Labor Day in September 1999. At my next appointment I found out I shouldn't wait much longer to set a date for surgery if I was thinking of having surgery at all. My doctor said the cancer was close to spreading out of my prostate and into the rest of my body. He told me the procedure I needed was called a "radical prostatectomy" (complete removal of the prostate).

I told my doctor I knew what the word *positive* meant but I needed a yes or no. He told me *yes,* I had cancer, which then hit me like a ton of bricks. He told me the type of cancer I had was adeno carcinoma and someone my age would do better having a radical prostatectomy because he would have a better chance of getting all the cancer. A few days later, wondering what to do, I talked with another doctor who told me the same thing. I talked with my wife again, and soon made the decision to go ahead with the operation.

My thoughts were running wild. What was I going to do? Was I going to die? And if so, how? Would my time remaining be a slow, agonizing, and painful existence and then death? I didn't know! And then my thoughts turned to family members. What was my wife thinking and feeling and was she as scared as I was or maybe worse? How would she finish raising our kids by herself on one income? Then my thoughts turned to our kids and how this was going to affect them. I was very concerned how it would affect them personally. Would they be angry, and if so, would they be angry at me? These were the things I was most concerned about. My mind was racing and I started becoming confused and depressed. Then I wondered about my mother and my siblings. What would my mother think when she found out about my cancer, knowing she had already lost her husband (my father) to another terrible disease? My siblings were older than me. I was the youngest, the baby of the family. I also wondered what their reactions would be after finding out their little brother had cancer. I knew my mother was getting older and I definitely didn't want to worry her. She had enough on her mind as it was. I needed to tell them and not keep it a secret.

I thought of my father, who had died many years before from amyotrophic lateral sclerosis (ALS), also called Lou Gehrig's disease. I was in my early teens when we started to notice his balance was unstable. He had gone to the Mayo Clinic for diagnosis and, as time went on, he started using a cane. He went from one cane to two canes within a couple of years as his disease got worse. He was a fighter, fighting his disease every step of the way and never giving up. This made me concerned what my kids would eventually remember about me and how my cancer would affect their lives as they finished growing up. They were young and impressionable, as I had been, and at a very critical time in their lives. If I died, or was sick from cancer and treatments, would they miss some of the better years getting to know their father as kids should? It was that part of my life that I missed while I was growing up. I felt, in a way, as if I was letting the whole family down and I was responsible for this nightmare I was thrown into.

My wife was wonderful and worked diligently on reading about prostate cancer and keeping me informed on all her findings. She also was helping me to stay positive and to remind me of what I was learning on my own about cancer. But at that point, she was the one keeping me informed, I was still in shock. Without her help I really don't know what might have happened or where I would be right now. I can now remember being too preoccupied about what was happening. I soon had to take some time off from my summer job as a tour guide and motor coach driver. I was worried about a possible accident as the cancer consumed my every thought. I just couldn't keep my mind on my touring and driving and would find myself in some kind of mental fog. A few of my close friends and coworkers knew, but I didn't tell most of them. Somehow I'm sure the word got out. As my surgery date was closing in on me fast, I also wondered what my family would do if I didn't make it through the surgery. All these things and more were consuming my every thought.

My surgery was on October 5, 1999, by two of the best urologists I could find in the state of Alaska. They came very highly recommended so I decided to go with them working together as a team. The surgery went well and a couple of days later, as I lay in the hospital recovering, one of my doctors told me the operation "went well" and they had removed the cancer.

Three days after my operation I was discharged from the hospital and went home. My wife noticed that the paperwork we received after the surgery didn't look quite right and immediately went to the hospital lab to talk with someone there about the results of the operation. At the lab a doctor told her they had not removed all the cancer and had actually cut through some of the cancer cells. They told her it was called "positive margins." Ever since that day, I knew there was an excellent chance of seeing my cancer return. From that moment on I became obsessed, really obsessed, with trying to find anything that might work in slowing or stopping the cancer. I was becoming frantic and wanted it all just to stop and go away. Maybe it was all a big nightmare and I just needed to wake up. But I knew this nightmare wasn't the kind that would go away. My doctor visits and my lab blood tests continued for years as did my self-education in this field. As time went on all my studying started paying off and started coming together on what I needed to do when the cancer started returning, if not sooner. *I was preparing myself for the fight of my life and the fight for my life!*

I spent evenings and weekends, sometimes staying up all night studying, trying to make sense out of what was happening. My search continued for years. My checkups went from a blood test every three months to every six months for nearly five years. Then, slowly, my PSA numbers started creeping back up, just a fraction at a time. I then returned to getting blood tests every three months.

In February 2005, I returned to my doctor to have another blood test, only to find my PSA numbers had tripled within a three-month period. These numbers were frightening and I knew then it was becoming serious. The next time I went in to see my doctor he finally recommended, "just a little radiation" would be the next best thing to do. At this very moment, I had to make another major decision to either stay with what my doctor was recommending or go for it on my own and put into play what I had learned. This is when I thought, "Most people would do exactly what their doctor recommended because what other choices do we have, right"? Well, I found out we do have other choices, so I started making them happen. I haven't looked back since and I'm feeling great. Take charge of your life and your health, *right now*, or you too may wind up with some kind of disease you really don't want to have. If you wait, the choices grow slim and you may not be able to change your health problem in time.

Again, I realized I had to make some very big sacrifices with the kind of foods I really loved. I needed to change my diet forever if I was going to beat the cancer that was slowly starting to grow and multiply in my body again. I found that you have to be on top of the cancer all the time and not think that just because you had an operation and just because your doctor said it's gone, that it was really gone for good. I kept thinking about the cancer diets and herbs and all the great nutritional products I was learning more and more about.

I had been wading through tons of scientific research about cancer, nutritional products, and the advantages of eating the right foods, as each year went by since my surgery. I knew I had to do something and it would have to be right now, if not sooner. I realized this was something that was not going away. I had already been watching what I was eating very closely but, as I got further and further away from my post surgery date, I started to slip a little with the sugar and carbohydrates, thinking it wouldn't make a difference if I ate the foods I liked once in a while. I was wrong and was once again feeding the cancer by what I was eating, although I was watching a little better than before.

According to my doctor, the radiation treatments and drugs would probably not stop or get rid of the cancer, they would only slow it down at best. From what I had learned, I now realized that the cancer was spreading through my whole body and had been the whole time. I was also learning more about prescription medications and the problems they can bring. I thought, "If I keep going ahead with this plan there may not be a way out." So, I was now ready to make my move and start my fight from what I had learned in the years since my operation.

I had heard very few good stories and a lot of horror stories about the effects of radiation on the body now and also later in life. So, being stubborn, but more educated in the field of nutrition by now, I decided to start a serious nutritional regimen instead of the radiation. My search continued throughout this time, and still continues today. The information and products I have found are incredible. I can now say, "My cancer is gone and my PSA levels are under control," which still sounds incredible every time I say it. Please read on and I will explain to you how I won my battle against cancer, the natural way.

I made a drastic decision to go off all the medication my doctor had given me which was not, according to my doctor, killing the cancer. If what I had learned about nutrition was going to work, now was the time to do it. I immediately changed my whole way of eating and started taking the products listed in this book, which I had learned would improve my body, and my immune system, and help fight my cancer.

When I went back to see my doctor for another PSA blood test, my numbers had dropped to half of what they had been three months earlier. I then knew, from that moment, that what I was doing was starting to work wonders, if not miracles. I knew if my PSA numbers continued to go down at the same rate for the next three months or so I would be doing extremely well and might be in the clear if I kept following my plan of attack.

When I went in for my next doctor's appointment another three months had gone by. After my PSA blood test I saw the doctor. When he came into the room he said, "Wow, the medicine you're taking must be working." That was when I told him I *had not* been taking my meds since for the past six months.

So you see, there is hope, and I know this now for sure. Having this proof of my PSA numbers going down was *fantastic* news. Most doctors would probably tell you, as mine did, "That just doesn't happen. PSA numbers don't go down by themselves," talking about a person with prostate cancer, or like me, post prostate cancer. Well my numbers didn't go down by themselves. They had help, a lot of help. The fact was that none of that help was from prescription drugs or radiation. All the help was from natural products from what I had learned about on my own. What this all means is, I beat the cancer I had and life has meaning once again. This is all because of what I've learned and the program I set for myself to follow and continue to follow today. Life *is* good, believe it!

More fantastic news came on July 13, 2005, when I went in for another three month blood test. I thought my PSA numbers had gone down more than the last time, but I was still very nervous. I had been following the strict cancer diet regimen that I had been on since my last test in the hopes that my PSA numbers would go down even more. Within fifteen minutes, the test results came back and my PSA numbers had fallen way down again. I was *ecstatic*, to say the least, and left the building jumping in the air and screaming, *"I did it!"* This proved to me again I was beating my cancer. I was now, hopefully, in the clear, and safe from any serious cancer onset in the future, as long as I stayed on top of it. It set in stone what I need to do if my cancer was ever to return.

A PSA blood test is not a sure sign of cancer and is not a cancer diagnosis. It can, and sometimes does, mean other problems are present. If your PSA numbers are low or high, it could mean you have prostatitis, (inflammation of the prostate). This condition is said to be benign (meaning no cancer). You could also have other types of infection. Studies have found almost 25% of men with a low PSA level can still have prostate cancer.

Have both a PSA blood test and a digital (finger) exam done if you think you're having problems. The digital can be embarrassing for some, which is one of the reasons why some men never go in to be checked, even when a problem does develop. Then, if needed, you can discuss a biopsy with your doctor. A biopsy, digital exam, and a PSA are the best ways to be sure if cancer is part of your life.

According to the American Cancer Society, African American men are more likely to have prostate cancer than any other ethnic group. White men are second in line and are most likely to contract prostate cancer when they are younger. This was me at age 48. Latino men are next, but are at a low risk. However, prostate cancer is the most common cancer among the Latino group. Asian and Native American men have the lowest risk among these groups.

NOTES

<u>NOTES</u>

PART 2

------◆------

CANCER MUST BE STOPPED

MOST CANCER AND DISEASE CAN BE STOPPED
IF CAUGHT IN TIME

One of the oldest descriptions of cancer was discovered in Egypt and dates back to around 1600 B.C. The word *cancer* is thought to have been created by Hippocrates, who is considered the "Father of Medicine" (460-370 B.C.). Some of the earliest evidence of cancer was found in fossilized bone tumors from human mummies in ancient Egypt and in ancient manuscripts. Now, in the 21st century, we have a better understanding of the damage cancer has done to our society. Rudolf Virchow, the founder of cellular pathology, was one of the few who paved the way for the modern study of cancer.

Now is the time to do some serious thinking about our approach to cancer and disease. It is time we looked directly at the prevention and elimination of cancer, not just the remission or a prescription for cancer. In recent times, some prescription drugs have cured some forms of cancer. However, there is still a lot of cancer killing many people. Data from various agencies such as the National Cancer Institute and others show that up to 90% of all cancers are products of our lifestyle, a lack of exercise, exposure to toxic chemicals, and what we choose to eat and drink. Many of us are consuming processed foods; foods and drinks high in artificial sweeteners and in processed sugars; foods high in carbohydrates and trans-fatty acids; and genetically engineered foods, (GEF). These types of foods, and many others that we think would be "healthy foods," also contain high amounts of toxic chemicals.

Most of us live in a fast-paced world. We look for a quick fix when things go wrong, and then go running to our doctors wondering how and why this could happen to us. When people initially find out they have a disease such as cancer, for many the world seems to end and sometimes depression sets in. Then most of us realize we have a choice to make—either get ready to die, or prepare to fight for our lives and live to see better days. It is when we realize this, and make a plan to fight, that cancer no longer controls our lives. I know. I'm living proof that a person can win the battle with cancer and disease with a positive attitude and an informed plan of action.

Research shows cancer does not have to be a death sentence. Cancer is our body screaming for immediate help. We have a choice to make. We can do this with prescription drugs, chemotherapy, radiation, and surgery, or with nutrition, herbs, the correct foods, exercise, and by keeping our bodies alkaline. People who don't have cancer, or another disease, rarely think about this growing problem until the day it comes knocking on their door. We've been conditioned over the years to leave our health in our doctor's hands and made to believe that our medical industry is making great discoveries in the field of cancer and other diseases. If you're waiting for the medical industry to work a miracle, it could cost you your life.

There are primary and secondary causes of disease. Cancer, above all other diseases, has countless secondary causes. The prime cause of cancer is the replacement of the respiration of oxygen by the fermentation of sugar. This means, all normal body cells meet their energy needs by respiration of oxygen. Cancer cells meet their energy needs, in great part, by fermentation (oxygen deficiency). In 1931 and 1944, Dr. Otto Warburg won Nobel prizes for his work in studying cancer. He said, "Cancer cannot live in an oxygen-rich environment." Years later, two-time Nobel Prize winner, Linus Pauling, Ph.D., had this to say regarding our cancer industry: "Everyone should know that most cancer research is largely a fraud and that the major cancer research organizations are derelict in their duties to the people who support them."

Dr. John Bailer, who spent 20 years on the staff of the U.S. National Cancer Institute, had this to say about the American Cancer Society, "The five-year survival statistics are very misleading; they now count things that are not cancer, making patients appear to live longer." He went on to say, "Our whole cancer research in the last 20 years has been a total failure." I should mention that the "five-year survival time," mentioned above is the period of time your doctor may give you to be cancer free. Nowadays, this time frame is usually extended to seven years instead of five.

Cancer cells live in our bodies without harming us until our immune system gets run down and does not run properly. Our T cells kill the cancer cells, dissolving them constantly. Our normal cells are protected by an enzyme called Superoxide dismutase. Cancer cells go after the nitrogen produced from the protein in the muscle tissue. This can start the breakdown of our body's tissues over time. This breakdown of tissue is called cachexia and will waste a body away, causing it to become weaker and weaker until, finally, it dies. There are many things that can be done. Please keep reading.

Cancer cells are the result of damage done to our DNA in the cell's nucleus which turns our healthy cells into cancer cells. These cancerous cells start to grow much faster than our healthy cells. These cells then compete with our healthy cells for the nutrients needed as the cancer cells multiply out of control. These cancer cells then travel through our bodies and find weak areas to attach themselves to, and they can grow tentacles and tumors that reach out to invade other areas. Cancer develops anaerobic metabolisms and creates energy in the absence of oxygen.

Cancer cells also absorb blood sugar and glucose much faster than our healthy cells, and steal life-supporting energy from our noncancerous cells. Consequently, a person with cancer can also have weak noncancerous cells. According to studies, 40% of all cancer patients die because of malnutrition of these weakened cells alone. Some patients can be weakened to the point of being bedridden. If this happens to you because of conventional methods of treatment, and you can't keep anything in your stomach, sip small amounts of Noni juice from your health food store to help regain your strength. The taste of Noni juice takes getting used to but the juice is extremely healthy.

In 1936, the U.S. Senate issued Document No. 264 with information regarding the lack of minerals in our food and their relationship to good health. They reported that many diseases were caused by the depletion of our soils and that the soil no longer provided plants with enough mineral elements to keep us healthy. Today, it seems we are trading the minerals in our soils for pesticides and other chemicals. The chemicals we use keep building up in our soil over the years as more plants are harvested and more chemicals are used. Some of these chemicals take 100 years or more to break down before they are no longer detected in the soil.

PEOPLE SPEAK OUT
ABOUT OUR HEALTH INDUSTRY

I question why our government doesn't recognize or acknowledge the great advancements health and nutrition research companies are making in this field, and work with them until cancer is cured. Maybe the problem is that they do recognize this and are wondering what might happen if people started to cure themselves. It seems to me, the more I learn about our big industries, the more I believe it's all about money, big money.

Today world governments, along with the U.S. government, are trying to regulate our consumption of nutritional products and take them from us, right off the shelves as they already have in Australia and other countries. I know this sounds crazy, and you may think this information is wrong. Well, it's not wrong. Believe me when I say this. Go to: *www.saveoursupplements.org* to see how you can help. This is happening right now. Or look at the end of this book under "Save Our Supplements."

We would be much further ahead if the medical and nutritional fields worked together, hand in hand, but less than 1% of the National Cancer Institute budget is devoted to nutrition studies, and even that small amount had to be forced on the Institute by a special amendment of the National Cancer Act in 1974. Pharmaceutical companies can't make big money in the production of natural products, so very little money, if any, is used for research in this field.

*A 1986 report in the New England Journal of Medicine said, "Some 35 years of intense effort focused largely on improving treatment must be judged a qualified failure." The report went on to say, "We are losing the war against cancer", and argued for a shift in emphasis towards **prevention**, if there is to be substantial progress.*

Our medical and nutritional products are, and have been, suppressed in our society by current laws, regulations, and policies. The problems we are now having in our health industry are the result. Now, an interest in alternative medicine is on the rise. Some agencies in our government are trying to stop nutritional supplements from being sold, and put them in the hands of the Federal Drug Administration (FDA), American Medical Association (AMA), or similar government departments, to be monitored.

Benjamin Rush, a famous doctor in colonial America, and a signer of the Declaration of Independence, wrote: "The Constitution of this Republic should make special provision for medical freedom as well as religious freedom. To restrict the art of healing to one class of men and deny equal privilege to others will constitute the Bastille of medical science. All such laws are un-American and despotic." He also said "Unless we put medical freedom into the Constitution, the time will come when medicine will organize itself into an undercover dictatorship." What great statements these were in his day. And now look what's happening today.

Senator Paul Douglas of Illinois declared on the Senate floor on December 6, 1963, "It's a terrible thing that we cannot really trust either the FDA or the National Cancer Institute (NCI).

According to Irwin Zimen, M.D., a professor of medicine at UCLA College of Medicine, "the use of food as a drug had always been important until the modern drug industry arose in the 19th century." Prior to World War II, many herbs used by the U.S. Pharmacopoeia, which is the official listing of accepted medicines, were listed side by side with the chemical drugs being used at that time.

In the March 22, 2004 edition of Fortune magazine, in an article by Dr. Clifton Leaf called, "Why we are losing the war on cancer, and how to win it," he described today's cancer research as "dysfunctional" because of the bureaucracy of the FDA that stands in the way of research and the goals of the researchers. He went on to say these kinds of obstacles forced them to only look at the smallest improvements within the same methods that were already not working. If a particular drug shrinks a tumor by 10% and increases a patient's life by five months it is considered a success. The scientists and physicians doing the research are then rewarded for academic achievement and publication rather than for new discoveries, ideas, or methods. The FDA will then push through new medications faster if they are similar to the approved methods already in place.

Dr. Leaf said cancer research is a business. If the methods are not profitable, they are not researched. This is why natural methods of treatments and *prevention* are not researched, because they are not profitable for the medical field and pharmaceutical industry. So, cancer research is at a standstill compared to the other areas of scientific research. Meanwhile, what happens to the people in need that think our government and the FDA are really doing their best in the fight against cancer?

An article called, "How cancer politics have kept you in the dark regarding successful alternatives," was written by John Diamond, M.D., and Lee Cowden, M.D. In the fourth paragraph they said, "Money leads politics by the nose. The financial interests of drug companies, conventional cancer doctors, hospitals, HMOs and others in what is known as the Cancer Establishment, have eclipsed the integrity of the Hippocratic Oath; money and politics have proclaimed conventional approaches as scientifically validated and therefore mandated by law. The terrible flaw in the convenient financial setup is that the profits that flow to the cancer establishment are derived from human lives lost to cancer because successful alternative approaches are outlawed or unreported." The rest of this article can be found at: www.whale.to/w/politic.html.

A study commissioned in 2004 by the "Dietary Supplement Education Alliance," found that nutritional supplements such as folic acid and calcium could cut billions of dollars in health care costs over the next five years. This study came out of the House Subcommittee on Human Rights and Wellness. The results showed calcium supplements could prevent 734,000 hip fractures in the 65-and-over ages, which could save $13.9 billion. The use of folic acid could prevent neural tube birth defects and save $11.3 billion in lifetime costs by preventing around 3,000 of these birth defects. These are only two of all the very important supplements our bodies need each and every day to stay healthy. Just think what *could* happen if we started using more supplements!

Dr. Mercola, a well known physician and natural health care expert, is the author of the world's most popular natural health newsletter, *www.mercola.com*. Dr. Mercola shared his thoughts about the medical industry. He said, "The conventional medical paradigm has been a destructive influence in our culture, promoting disease by pinning all focus on mere treatments that patch over existing illness while virtually ignoring both prevention and real cure. By far, the key contributor to this dangerous misperception of what health care means is the pharmaceutical industry. The drug companies thrive in a state where people remain sick and more are getting sick, as that means both repeat customers and a growing base for their overpriced treatments." He went on to say through his report that drug companies generate hundreds of billions of dollars in profit annually. This enormous amount of capital has created the largest legislative lobbying influence in Congress. If you would like to read this whole report, go to: *www.mercola.com/forms/myvision.htm*.

In 2004, Dan Burton, chairman of the House Government Reform Subcommittee on Human Rights and Wellness, held a hearing entitled "Dietary Supplements: Nature's Answer to Cost-Preventive Medicine." In this hearing, he focused on a preventive role in individual health care. In part of his statement he said, "I, along with millions of Americans, firmly believe that dietary supplements have been shown through credible scientific research and historical use to be of immeasurable benefit to human health. I believe, when used responsibly, and in consultation with a primary care physician, these products can greatly enhance an individual's overall personal health."

Presently, the medical society does not look upon nutritional supplements as a means to improve our health. Some people now believe that man-made medicines from laboratories, and not nature, are the right answers for all our health problems. But, even today, about 50% of the most commonly used prescribed drugs are made from a plant source (herb) or an imitation of a plant source.

Stop here for a minute and think. Take a deep breath and let in some oxygen. Get used to breathing deep to let in extra oxygen. Please remember, I am not a doctor, but I am living proof that I won my personal war with cancer "the natural way" without drugs and dangerous therapies when my cancer came back, more aggressively, four years after my surgery. How I did this is what this book is all about. If just one person survives cancer or disease, and can live a healthy, productive life by learning from this book, my effort in writing this book will have been very worthwhile for both of us. Please take another deep breath and read on.

Cancer, as of 2002, is the number one killer disease in the world, moving cardiovascular (heart) disease into second place. Cancer is also the leading cause of death in children between the ages of 3 and 14. The startling truth is that more and more people, young and old, are developing this disease. By the end of this century, 50% of us or more are expected to develop cancer. Where is it going to stop? It happened to me at age 48, prostate cancer to be exact, and it can also happen to you. Not only prostate cancer but breast cancer, in both genders, and all the other types of cancer and disease are waiting to cripple or destroy you, if you give them half a chance. So, don't give them a chance! Start fighting now.

It has been more than 30 years of research and development of new drugs since President Nixon gave his speech on winning the war on cancer. Since then the death toll from cancer has still risen 73%, which is 1.5 times greater than the U.S. population growth. The number of people who die every day from cancer is the same as one World Trade Center collapsing every day. Doctors are now recommending that men have a PSA as early as age 35 and women should have a mammogram by 40 years of age. Cancer is now becoming a disease for younger men and women and not just for the older generation. One out of every two men, and two out of every three women, will develop some form of cancer in their lifetime in this century, not to mention a multitude of other diseases. Start to learn about preventing these diseases by learning about nutrition.

Another study by the Harvard Medical School and the Public Citizens, a consumer advocacy organization, was published in the Journal of the American Medical Association (AMA). The study reported 20% of all new drugs are found to have serious or life-threatening adverse effects on the body which are unknown or undisclosed. Within seven years after a drug is first introduced into the U.S. marketplace, half of all serious adverse effects are detected, such as damage to the heart, liver, bone marrow, and risks with pregnancy. To read more about this, go to the reference pages and look for "Poison for Profit" and "Alert."

In *A Cancer Battle Plan Sourcebook*, David Frahm, said, "Relying on pharmaceutical drugs is like putting Band-Aids on skin cancer: Drugs mask symptoms and divert attention from dealing with underlying causes." He went on to say, "Medicinal drugs rob the body of nutrients and thus weaken its self-healing and protective systems."

Cancer is a systemic disease. Something has weakened our system, allowing the cancer cells we all have naturally accruing in our body to thrive. Once a tumor is an actually detectable cancer, cells have already spread throughout the entire body. When the goal is to strengthen the body so it can heal itself, it doesn't matter where in the body the cancer may be.

Prescription medications can be dangerous and are acidic to the body. They are also foreign to the body and can, in turn, block the absorption of nutrients. James Balch, M.D., said, "All drugs are potentially dangerous," and "The more drugs you take, and the longer you take them, the more likely you are to be nutritionally deficient."

An article in the April 15, 1998 edition of *USA Today* says, "Drug reactions kill 100,000 patients a year." In this number, there were no medications that had been prescribed incorrectly or given to the wrong patients. These were pharmaceutical prescriptions prescribed by trained medical physicians for correctly diagnosed problems. That's a big number of people to be so incorrectly diagnosed.

As the science of nutritional supplements grows, researchers learn more and more about how all nutrients work together with the body. Taking just a few vitamins or minerals is better than none, but doesn't work as well as taking a whole food supplement.

Whole food supplements can offset the need for other nutrients not being taken or absorbed correctly. Taking supplements together in the right strengths can make an enormous difference. That's why a whole food supplement is an excellent way to go. It has everything in the right proportions and can be absorbed more easily by the body. A good whole food vitamin in liquid form can be up to 500% more bio-available (usable) to the body than hard vitamins, and a lot easier to swallow. That's why I take a whole food supplement every day. There is more on this later.

The reference pages in the back of this book aren't just to back up what I have written here. They are also a study guide for me to fall back on and for you to use to find out about good health. Make sure you take the time to go through the reference pages and websites carefully.

OUR LIVES ARE UNDER STRESS

Most people today live in the fast lane, with high-stress jobs and a high-stress home life, where both parents must work to pay the bills. Parents send their kids home to an empty house to fix their own unhealthy meals of processed foods full of preservatives, high in salt, sugar, fat, and trans-fatty acids, to be swallowed down with an ice cold pop or juice filled with sugar or dangerous artificial sweeteners. Now is the time to act and live a healthy life. Disease doesn't happen overnight. It takes years, and it will also take years off your life before you know it.

Stress can be overwhelming and very intense, putting a terrible burden on your health and life. If you don't rid yourself of stress by exercising regularly, eating right, and supplementing your body with the best nutritional products available, your lifestyle may lead to an early grave. Stress not only gives some of us headaches, heartburn, and chronic fatigue, but may lead to life-threatening disease such as cancer.

Stress can prevent absorption of many nutrients and uses them up much faster, leaving your body depleted of vital nutrients. This can cause many problems. It can stress out the immune, adrenal, and digestive systems as gastrointestinal distress sets in along with depression, anxiety, and a lack of desire. Stress can be very dangerous, and I sincerely believe it played a big part in my getting cancer.

Nutritional supplements are very important for combating stress. One of them is Omega 3, which helps with amino acids in the body. Stress can open the door to disease by acting as a precursor to other illnesses. When your immune system is weak from stress and a lack of nutritional supplements, you usually start by feeling run down. You catch colds, flu, your joints hurt, and your white blood cell count goes way down, often leaving you unable to fight off illnesses. Your body starts to shut down. The adrenal system, hypothalamus, pituitary, and the thyroid have much more stress put on them. This problem needs to be corrected with exercise, nutritional supplements, and a wholesome diet in order to put your body back in the healthy range.

Acute stress stimulates the production of adrenaline, whereas cortisol is the hormone of chronic stress. Too much of either of these hormones increases the possibility of cardiovascular disease and the onset of other types of disease. Too much adrenaline for too long a time can cause arterial spasms, and even rupture of heart muscle fibers. Too much cortisol can raise cholesterol and cause a loss of potassium and other essential minerals. All this, over time, can lead to a run down immune system, leaving your body susceptible to other diseases.

Breathe deeply, and let the oxygen in. Do this several times a day whether you feel stressed or not. Get more oxygen into your system and it can help prepare itself for the next stressful situations. Also, laugh and think positively. These two positive things can work miracles in the body.

Make it a point to watch the DVD "What the Bleep Do We Know!?" Our bodies are more than 70% water. Pay particular attention to the photos showing what a change in our body energy, attitude, and thoughts can do to a drop of water. Then decide what you want your body fluid to look like.

<u>NOTES</u>

NOTES

PART 3

SOME VERY IMPORTANT BASICS

EXERCISE IS A MUST

Regular exercise is always *extremely* important for the young and old, whether fighting stress, disease, or cancer, and is a must just for good physical health. It is true that, "if you don't use it, you lose it." Fewer than 20% of adult Americans engage in regular exercise, and 55% are said to be inadequately active. The remaining 30% fit into the couch potato category. Being overweight is one of the leading causes of adult onset of diabetes and several kinds of cancer. Starting an exercise routine will start you on your way to becoming much healthier, and please don't say you're too busy.

Exercise is a great way to better your health. It is also one of the few ways to cleanse your lymphatic system, especially when fighting cancer and disease. There is an easy exercise called *rebounding*. Rebounding is jumping up and down on a small inside, or larger outside, trampoline. This causes g-forces to create the gravitational pull necessary to positively stimulate almost every cell in the body and help remove lymphatic fluids, which are filled with metabolic toxic waste. The body dumps this waste into its bloodstream where it is eventually removed from the body. This waste can include cancerous cells, fat, viruses, and heavy metals such as lead, mercury, aluminum, and so forth.

If you're looking for a magic pill that will keep you healthy, I have some bad news for you—there is no such pill. A professor of nutrition an epidemiology at the Harvard School of Public Health has said, "Good nutrition is essential for health" and "The single thing that comes close to a magic pill, in terms of its benefits, is exercise." Exercise has positive effects against many serious diseases.

I believe I have won my battle with cancer, not because of what my doctor told me, but from what I have learned on my own about exercise, nutritional products, herbs, and a special cancer diet I have followed very closely. You will see by reading this book, that I do believe in what my doctor says, but I also realize doctors are professionals usually trained only in the field they specialize in, just like most of us. We are trained as professionals, but usually only in the field we work in.

We usually get more than one opinion before having a major repair done to our home or automobile. We should be the same or better with our bodies. Many times we find that two specialists in the same field have very different opinions on how to fix the same problem. This usually causes us to do some independent research to try to decide which technique we want to use. Personal recommendations frequently help us choose which way we want to go. Please take a minute to think about that. This leads me to say again, "I am not a professional in the field of medicine or nutrition, but I have found a way of life that has rid my body of cancer."

OVERWEIGHT?

Too many fattening foods, for too many years, and all of a sudden you're fighting the fat hanging off your body. Studies show that from 1976 to 2000 obesity increased from 14.4% to 30.9% of the U.S. population. The fatter we get the higher our risk becomes of contracting all types of diseases. People are spending more money on meals away from home than ever before, feeding their families fatty processed foods with very few nutrients. A child with overweight parents has a 40% to 80% chance of being overweight and may have a stronger biological drive to eat. Too much of this type of food can also bring about diabetes.

Studies also show that 34% of adult women are obese in the United States compared to 28% of men, and women have a much harder time loosing the weight.

In 2003, the Center for Disease Control declared obesity the most important public-health issue in the United States. Obesity increases risks of cancer, type II diabetes and cardiovascular disease. Children and teenagers are seeing rapid increases in the onset of diabetes. A scary two-thirds of people living in the United States are now overweight or obese. Children who develop diabetes before the age of 14 can expect their lives to be reduced by 17 to 29 years. Look this up for yourself at *www.briancalkins.com*. Also check out this website on the Glycemic Index (GI) at *www.glycemicindex.com*.

Americans spend more than $33 million annually to find the magic weight loss pill. Fat, sugar, and yes, even diet drinks with artificial sweeteners are among the many contributing factors in excess weight, and weight (fat) that is lost is usually regained within a year. Obesity is the most common nutritional disorder in the world today and definitely in the United States. Obesity in our country has risen 65% in the past 10 years.

People believe they gain weight when they eat too much, and this is true, but why? A big part of *why* we are gaining weight so easily is the nutritionally deficient foods we are so obsessed with. The truth is, Americans today are nutritionally deficient people. The wrong types of food may fill your stomach but the body becomes hungry shortly after a meal because the foods eaten are without good nutrients and are called nutrient–deficient foods, dead foods, and junk foods. This is a serious problem and, without people knowing, it's leading us into many types of diseases.

One big reason for weight gain is having an acidic environment (pH) in your body. This is a huge factor in weight gain, obesity, diabetes and cancer. When your body is too acidic, large amounts of insulin are produced, which converts the calories into fat. It is said your body stimulates a genetic response to starvation and, in turn, stores the fat. This directly stimulates or impedes the insulin-glucagon axis, which makes the body produce extra insulin. It is said, the more insulin available (produced), the higher the probability that fat is produced rather than being used up as energy. When there is increased pressure to make extra insulin, the immune system over-responds with stress in the cells, which then makes it difficult for them to do their job and they burn out. This is another reason why acidosis is said to be a precursor to diabetes. This is a big reason why we must keep our bodies alkaline. An acid pH will also decrease oxygen in the blood, lead to disease and eventually cause death. Go to: *www.PeopleAgainstCancer.com*.

Gamma linolenic acid (GLA) can aid in weight loss. It is an omega-6 fatty acid, and is mainly found in borage and evening primrose oils. Read a little more about GLA later in this book. Omega-3 also aids in weight loss and is found mostly in Flax seed and fish oils. Omega-3 is associated with reduced heart disease and reduced fat storage by stimulating fat burning by increasing the body's metabolic rate. Omega-3 also contains two fatty acids that are found in fish. They are DHA and EPA and work excellently in preventing disease. It is said fish are now showing high levels of mercury, which is a toxic metal. Be careful of the type of fish you eat, where it is from, and where you buy it. These products are easily found at your local health food store.

Many people find it extremely hard to change their diet, even if it means their health will worsen if they don't lose weight. Other people just don't understand the impact that eating the wrong food has on their bodies over time. If you're unwilling to change, or find it extremely difficult, try this. The next time you go shopping, go to a health food store that sells groceries and a farmers market to buy fresh produce, vegetables, and free-range meats. Try eating more "live foods" that are full of nutrients. Your body will feel full, you won't have to eat as much to be full and you will remain full longer. Additionally, eat smaller portions and eat more slowly. You will then start to lose weight and, with exercise, just think what could happen. You can do it, and you will be amazed at the results.

If you want to feel better and not catch every cold or flu that comes along, and also increase your energy, buy fresh organic foods and start taking good nutritional supplements. If you can't do without your junk foods, buy them at your health food store without all the preservatives (chemicals), processed sugars, and processed flours. You may not know it, but preservatives are chemicals, chemicals are toxins, and many of these are poison, and poisonous to your body. These chemicals also keep your immune system run down to where your body has an extremely hard time keeping you healthy.

Believe it or not, roughly 90% to 95% of all man-made foods can have up to 300 chemicals (toxins) added to each product that don't have to be listed on the label. Do yourself a favor and support your local organic food market and your local health food store so they'll be around to keep you healthy.

If you want to find out if you're overweight and find out what your body mass index (BMI) is, go to *www.nhlbisupport.com/bmi/ bmicalc.htm*. I have learned there are only two good ways of keeping weight off your body for life. In this book, I talk a little about the importance of changing what you eat, which is your diet, and the importance of exercising every day, even if it's only a walk down the street to start with. Take a long hard look at your eating habits and don't always eat just because you're hungry. When you do eat, eat something healthy. This food will stay with you longer and you won't feel as hungry later. Healthy foods will keep you full longer because of their nutritional value. Check out the spirulina ginseng balls I talk about later. They are an excellent source of food, full of protein, great for a snack, and will fill you up.

Keep a record of what you eat. Write everything down to see what you are eating. You will learn how to cut out the bad foods, change your eating habits and start eating more wisely. If you're fighting disease, you must get off all sugars, artificial sweeteners, processed foods, trans-fatty acids, processed flours, and refined carbohydrates (carbs). Check out the websites in the reference pages. This website will help you understand the difference in carbs. Go to: *www.briancalkins.com/simplevscomplexcarb.htm* and look around this same site for more great information.

To go further into better health, as you read through this book you will learn how to start detoxifying your body. You will also find other very important ways to improve your health and keep good health habits. If you do these things, watch out—you'll have more energy, lose weight, and feel much better. Wow, what a concept. You don't have to do all this at once, but you do have to get serious about it and do it within a reasonable amount of time and stick to it. By becoming involved with your health, you will become healthier and you could be saving yourself from crippling diseases such as arthritis, heart problems, diabetes, multiple sclerosis, cancer, and others. You might just stop an onset of one of these diseases earlier than you think. Also, think of the money you'll save on medical bills. Initially, organic foods may be an additional expense until you're used to eating healthier and know what to buy. After a while the costs will even out and you won't be spending much more money, if any. Just think of the junk foods you won't have to buy when you start to adjust to eating what your body really needs. Also consider the prescription medicine, doctor and hospital bills that could disappear or become a lot less expensive when you start to feel better. And if you still think you're spending more money, that's ok, you're worth it. If you have cancer, as I did, it's really not a question at all. It's a new way of life and a much, much healthier path to follow.

OUR WATER

Our bodies are mostly water and we need plenty of pure water each day to stay healthy and flush toxins out of our systems. Drinking other products in place of water will not flush the toxins out, so don't try and fool yourself. We need pure water that is as free of chlorine, fluoride, lead, and other toxic chemicals as possible.

The human body is 70% water and our blood is 90% water, so the quality and quantity of water you drink is crucial to your overall health. A whopping 75% of you are chronically dehydrated, and in 40% of you, your thirst mechanism is so weak you often mistake thirst for hunger. So, what do you do? You run out and "super-size" your next meal and swallow it down with an extra large soda. I used to think "That would really taste great," but that's not me today. I don't miss this type of eating, nor do I have any cravings for it anymore. Try replacing that large pop with bottled water since that's the kind they have for sale at most drive-up places. This way you won't be drinking city water with added chemicals.

Statistics show drinking at least five glasses of water a day will decrease by 45%, your risk of colon cancer and other ailments such as asthma, allergies, arthritis, and general body stiffness, to mention but a few. Let your water faucet run at least one minute before drinking from it to clear away some of the harmful chemicals and other residues. Chlorine, aluminum fluoride, and lead are some of the additives we drink in our water across the United States when we turn our faucets on. These additives can, and will add serious long-term consequences to your life and health. Although chlorine is a poison, it is added to water to kill bacteria and other living organisms.

There is one critical point here that might slip past us. Our bodies are living organisms that need good, clean water. But without chlorine to kill these germs, we could also be in trouble with the other additives that come from our pipes and into our glasses of water. One or more of the following comes out of our water pipes: copper, rust, pipe joint compounds, microscopic growths, viruses, arsenic, and diseases such as typhoid and cholera. Some, or all of the above come out of your home faucets, even if your water is considered clean. We do need a better system to bring our water to the table so we don't have to worry about what we're drinking, or if we're going to get sick or contract a disease. Aluminum fluoride is frequently added to our water to make it clear to see through. Fluoride is one of the most toxic and dangerous chemicals we know of and is like a time bomb in our bodies, according to Dr. Herbert Schwartz, chemist and biologist.

According to the U.S. Council of Environmental Quality, "Cancer risk among people drinking chlorinated water is 93% higher than among those whose water does not contain chlorine."

Joseph Price M.D., and doctor of internal medicine, wrote a controversial book called, Coronaries/Cholesterol/Chlorine. He says that, "it is a fact that the basic cause of arteriosclerosis, heart attacks, and stroke is chlorine."

Dr. Robert Carlson, Ph.D., professor of Biological Science at Kent State University, and respected researcher at the University of Minnesota says, "Chlorine is the greatest crippler and killer of modern times." Go to:

www.waterwarning.com/chlorinefact.htm.

Women with breast cancer show 60% higher levels of chlorination by-products in their breast tissues than women without breast cancer. Also, when we use steam rooms supplied with chlorinated water we inhale up to 50 times higher levels of chlorine because of the vaporization of water used for steam. Studies are now showing fluoride in our water does cause cancer. It also causes obesity by slowing down our metabolism, birth defects, thyroid problems, and prenatal deaths.

The book *Definitive Guide to Cancer* points out that fluoride can produce cancer, transforming normal human cells into cancerous ones, even at concentrations of only 1 PPM (part per million). Lab tests done on animals show, even at low doses, that the animals died before the test was over when aluminum fluoride was used. Researchers at the University of Texas studying the effects of fluoride on humans say, "The terrifying conclusion of the studies was that fluoride greatly induced cancer tumor growth." Read *A Cancer Battle Plan Sourcebook* by Dave Frahm. This is another excellent book. Always think before you drink.

Believe it or not, good, fresh water is also the best treatment for fluid retention. When you get less water than you need, your body will hold on to what water it does have. This can show up as swollen feet and hands. If you give yourself the amount of water you really need, only then will your body release its stored water. Water helps with weight loss, helps with proper muscle tone, helps the body function properly, and flushes out waste products. As a minimum, a person should drink eight ounces of water eight times a day, about two quarts. However, it is recommended an overweight person needs an additional eight ounces for every 25 pounds of excess weight. Also, increase your water intake as needed when exercising. Check out: *colon health.net/free_reports/h2oartcl.htm.*

Drinking distilled water is another story. Dr. Masaru Emoto is a doctor of alternative medicine and has done extensive research on water around the planet. He says all distilled water has lost its "inner order" while natural healthy water has not. He goes on to say, "Although this view is somewhat controversial, I am firmly convinced distilled water is harmful to our health." One of the biggest reasons is that distilled water is highly acidic and most people who eat the American diet are too acidic already (more on acidity later). Distilled water will also leach beneficial minerals from our bodies. While some think distilled water may be beneficial for a short time while detoxifying the body, it is counterproductive in the long run.

Cold water has been shown to absorb into your system faster than warm water. Other studies recommend drinking water at room temperature when drinking large amounts. If you're a marathon runner, or someone who works out heavily, drink small to medium amounts of water and wait until you're finished exercising before you drink a large amount. Otherwise, you may thin your blood by drinking too much water while over exerting and become ill. Drinking large amounts of cold liquid just before, during, or right after exercising can cause stomach cramps. When you do get the proper amount of water your body needs, your fluids will be in perfect balance and your body will then function better. When you live out of town and have your own water well, you are much further ahead in having good, fresh water to drink. Make sure it's clean and fresh by having your well water checked by a professional for possible chemicals you don't need to be drinking. Water is the magic potion for life, so make sure you get your fair share to drink daily.

Water is classified by the FDA in different categories. These are: spring waters, mineral waters, purified waters, sparkling waters, artesian waters, and well water.

Good alkaline water neutralizes acidity which, in turn, will help flush waste products out of the body. Water will help prevent and cure all kinds of diseases. A good book to read is *Your Body's Many Cries for Water* by F. Batmanghelidj, M.D.

A couple of good water filters that you might want to check into are Code Blue and Brita water filters. These filters should filter out close to everything except chlorine and fluoride, which means you shouldn't use it if you're filtering city water. These are good filters to use if you're not hooked up to city water or community water wells and have a water source where no chemicals are added and will fit in your refrigerator easily. If you want to filter out everything, you need to turn to the professionals or check the bigger varieties that can be installed in your home water line system. Otherwise, find a store that sells filtered water. Don't take this lightly and keep drinking water with chemical additives. It's your life. Try to be as healthy as you can.

ALKALINE AND ACIDIC BODIES

Our bodies are alkaline by nature, but become acidic by what we put in it. Maintaining an alkaline body is essential for life and health. Biochemists and medical physiologists recognize that our pH (parts of Hydrogen or potential Hydrogen) balance is one of the most important requirements of a healthy body, and is critical in our everyday life. Keeping our body's alkalinity in check is like investing in the future, your future health to be exact.

The explanation of disease comes down to two words, *"acid/alkaline imbalance."* Being overacidic can become a dangerous condition and will start to weaken our immune systems, leading to disease. Balancing our pH is a major step toward healing our bodies and maintaining better health.

You must keep your body's pH in balance. That balance is between 6.8 and 7.8. Normal blood functioning takes place between 7.36 and 7.44 with acidosis (too much acid) starting below 7.1. If you're fighting cancer or another disease, you *must* take a more aggressive approach and keep your pH at least 7.5 or higher. The lower the pH reading, the more acidic and oxygen-deprived your fluids are. An acidic state in your body will decrease the body's ability to repair cells that have been damaged and will decrease your chance of detoxifying your body properly. This, in turn, will make you much more susceptible to illnesses and fatigue.

Our bodies constantly neutralize acidic fluids to keep our systems working at their best. If we stay acidic, the body no longer neutralizes our acid wastes and starts to deposit these wastes in our tissues and organs. This, in itself, is a direct link to degenerative diseases such as diabetes, tuberculosis, osteoporosis, high blood pressure, lupus, heart disease, obesity, neurological problems, cancer, immune deficiencies and more. On the other hand, high alkalinity can also cause many of the same problems when our bodies remain at extremely high alkalinity levels for too long a period, which, fortunately, most of us do not have to worry about.

If you're keeping your alkalinity high to fight disease, make sure to check with you naturopathic doctor or another specialist in this field. Most diseases we call "old-age diseases" are actually lifestyle diseases caused by acidosis (too much acid), the lack of proper nutritional supplements, and what we choose to eat and drink. Start eating an alkaline diet of raw foods and remember your water. The alkalinity of water is a measure of how much acid the water can neutralize. If needed, go back a few pages and read the section on water again.

The concept of acid/alkaline imbalance as the cause of disease is not something new. In 1933, a New York physician, William Howard Hay, published a ground-breaking book, *A New Health Era*, in which he maintained all disease is caused by autotoxication (self-poisoning) due to acid accumulation in the body. More recently, in the book *Alkalize or Die*, Dr. Theodore A. Baroody, N.D., D.C., Ph.D., said essentially the same thing. He said, "The countless names of illnesses do not really matter. What does matter is that they all come from the same root cause, too much tissue acid waste in the body."

Acid/alkaline imbalance is becoming a very big problem at this point in the American diet. Our diets are way too high in acid-producing animal products, and far too low in alkaline-producing foods such as fresh vegetables and fruits. We also eat large amounts of acid-forming foods such as fried foods, white flour, processed sugar, and we drink acid-producing beverages such as coffee and soda pop. Checking our saliva or urine every few days is an excellent way to measure our overall pH levels. A simple test strip (pH paper) can be purchased at a health food store or drugstore and can help you find out what your pH is. You can substantially cut your risk of disease by balancing your body's pH, eating the right foods, using nutritional supplements and drinking the correct amounts of water every day. This is a very big part of our health problems in America today.

An acid pH decreases the amount of oxygen in the blood that is delivered to our cells. This makes our normal cells *very* unhealthy, which makes the body sluggish and can lead to disease, as I mentioned in the section on overweight. Essential life functions become inactive, which

can lead to a heart attack. Other problems can develop such as:
1. All forms of cancer
2. Immune deficiency
3. High blood pressure
4. High cholesterol
5. Strokes
6. Heart attacks
7. Dementia
8. Senility
9. Parkinson's Disease
10. Multiple Sclerosis
11. ALS
12. Diabetes
And the list goes on. If you don't think you need to be eating healthy, read this again.

MINERALS

Dr. Linus Pauling once said, "Every sickness, disease, and ailment can be traced back to a mineral deficiency."

Minerals are essential in the proper functioning of our bodies. Laboratory tests prove most of us are suffering deficiencies from the diets we eat, and our bodies are badly deficient in minerals due to the poor condition of the soils that grow our plants. Very few people get all the 60 plus minerals they need on a daily basis. Since we do not produce minerals on our own, we must get them from our food source. A deficiency of just one or more minerals can thus have a devastating effect on the body and, over time, can lead to poor health and disease, which may shorten our lives. Our fruits, vegetables, and grains no longer contain the right amount of minerals, no matter how much we eat, because of our depleted soils.

In 1992, a report by the Earth Summit Report said there is a severe decline in nutritional minerals in farm and range soils. This report talks about the worldwide decline and depletion of minerals in our soil, and was broken down by continents to show the percentages of each. The report showed Australia at 55% depletion, Africa at 74%, and the worst was North America at 85% depletion. We desperately need to bring our soils back into proper mineral balance. This may be the biggest reason why we need nutritional supplements in our diets today. A deficiency in only one mineral for example, can cause disease in our bodies and start to dissolve our bones to insure adequate mineral replacement. This can cause serious complications, if not corrected. When we lack vitamins, the body makes use of some of the minerals we get from the foods we eat. When we lack an intake of some basic minerals and important trace minerals, some of the vitamins become useless to the body's daily functions. This is one good reason minerals are so important in our everyday diet. Minerals make the world go around for all living creatures.

The differences in minerals can be deceiving, but are extremely important to us in our daily lives. *Metallic* minerals are nothing more than finely crushed-up rocks our bodies use very little of, are extremely hard to digest, and can be toxic. *Colloidal* minerals are those that have not yet been converted into a form to be used by the human body. They have bypassed the plant and are taken directly out of the ground. These may cause health problems. Research shows some colloidal mineral particles are larger in size than others. In this case, it is important to always find out where the product comes from and how it is processed.

Ionic minerals, which are smaller in size than other types of processed minerals, are found in a naturally occurring form in plants after the plant has used the minerals from the soil to grow. These minerals are extremely small in size, up to 10,000 times smaller than colloidal mineral particles. They come from organic sea or land vegetation, are free from contaminants and are the easiest minerals for our bodies to digest. Eating the correct food is extremely important for good health. We should be eating whole foods (live food) from plant sources, or getting our nutrients from good-quality whole food supplements.

Dr. Carl Reich discovered in the 1950s that many of his patients were curing themselves of degenerative diseases by taking over the recommended daily allowance (RDA) of calcium, magnesium, vitamin D and other nutrients he had suggested for them to take. He prescribed megadoses of minerals and vitamins to patients he was seeing in his practice. He went on to cure thousands by the 1980s. He finally lost his license for simply explaining that the consumption of minerals could prevent disease. It was too simple and not accepted in the medical and pharmaceutical communities.

Dr. C. Everett Koop had this to say in his 1988 Surgeon General's report to the U.S. Congress. "The top 10 causes of death in the U.S. are diet-related degenerative diseases. 94% of deaths in America could be directly linked to degenerative diseases that resulted from nutritional deficiency."

That pretty much says it all, wouldn't you think? It's time to wake up and "smell the nutrients" before it's too late, folks. Get involved with your health and give your body what it really needs. I encourage you to take a stand *now*, and start reading to find out how you can keep your body healthy, long-term.

SUNLIGHT AND VITAMIN D

Yes, we do need our sunshine! Sixty years or more of research shows exposure to natural sunlight decreases our incidence of cancer. That's right. The evidence is out. After years and years of avoiding the sun, and people actually hiding from it, our researchers are saying that we need it. Our chances are far greater of dying from a deficiency of vitamin D than of dying from skin cancer from the sun. Tests show colon, prostate, and breast cancers have a lower risk of cancerous lesions when vitamin D is present. A study from Finland also confirmed a connection with a deficiency of vitamin D and prostate cancer. There is also evidence showing autoimmune diseases such as type I diabetes (juvenile or insulin dependent), and rheumatoid arthritis can be caused by a lack of this vitamin.

People living in northern hemispheres, where the days are dark most of the winter months, could benefit from taking a vitamin D supplement. Don't forget about also taking a whole food supplement to get all your daily requirements of all the essential nutrients. You can find vitamin D combined with a good calcium and magnesium supplement. Seasonal affective disorder (SAD) is a major problem in colder climates where a lack of sun plays a big role in people's lives.

Studies show, when you are in the sun, people with a darker complexion than those who are lighter in complexion get about 50% less sun penetration. It takes about an hour of skin exposure to the sun for a dark-skinned person to make the same amount of vitamin D as it takes a light-skinned person to make in 10 to 15 minutes.

Over exposure to sun, and sunburn are major problems today and cause over one million new cases of skin cancer a year. This is what we have to watch out for. Small amounts of sun exposure, two to three times a week at 10 to 15 minutes a day, are said to be sufficient for 80% to 90% exposure of your skin. If you're with someone with darker skin who doesn't burn as easily as you, make sure you watch your skin and get out of the sun before you burn. Your body does not make too much vitamin D, even if you stay in the sun longer than you should. But you *can* consume too much vitamin D in pill form, so study up on vitamin D and always read the labels. It takes about one hour in the sun for your body to naturally make 20,000 IU of this very essential vitamin.

METABOLIC TYPES AND BLOOD TYPES

Learning your "metabolic type" is important in managing your health. This means fine-tuning your daily diet for your body type. By eating the right foods for your particular body type, you will clear up a lot of your aches and pains. Dr. Joseph Mercola, author of *The Total Health Program*, says your body has a unique bio-chemistry requiring certain proportions and types of healthy carbohydrates, fats, and proteins that differ from other people's. Some people require more protein and others require smaller amounts of carbohydrates to stay healthy. Your success with your diet may depend on your metabolic type. By learning your specific type, you will help fight and prevent disease, avoid premature aging and help achieve, and keep your ideal weight.

Another great book is, *Eat Right For Your Type*, by Dr. Peter D'Adamo. I also strongly recommend another book by this same author, *Cancer, Fight It with the Blood Type Diet*. These two books talk about the four blood types (A, B, AB, and O) and four diets for staying healthier, fighting cancer, living longer, achieving your ideal weight without starving, and becoming familiar with the types of food your body needs for *your* blood type. He says, "The secret to healthy, vigorous, and disease-free living might be as simple as knowing your blood type." This book shows that everyone should not be eating the same foods. The foods we absorb also have an impact on how our bodies handle stress according to our particular blood type. The pluses and minuses that go with each blood type are not significant, only the four major letter categories, A, B, AB, and O.

The book explains that each of the four blood types requires different food choices, contains information that allows you to make choices about what you should and should not be eating and drinking, and tells why these food choices have an effect on your health. If you're an O blood type, as I am, you should be avoiding wheat, corn, and a high carbohydrate intake.

This book has helped my wife and me clear up allergy problems we were having with certain types of foods that we should not have been eating. It talks about childhood illnesses, diabetes, and digestive problems. It also mentions the lectin-cancer connection, and shows why lectin agglutinates (clumps together). Excessive blood fats increase the production of fibrinogen, which also causes blood cells to get sticky and start clumping together, forming blood clots. Whereas eating saturated fats (oils) increases the chance of blood clots forming, a diet emphasizing polyunsaturated fats has the opposite effect. Lecithin may help with this problem. Also, check out the section on lecithin in this book. Don't get lectin and lecithin mixed up.

<u>NOTES</u>

NOTES

PART 4

———◆———

ARTIFICIAL AND NATURAL SWEETENERS AND REFINED SUGARS

SODA POP AND SUGAR

What about soda pop, you might ask? Let's first talk about regular pop, the stuff with sugar in it. Well, my friends, your health is at risk. Soda pop (cola) is full of processed sugar (about 12 to 15 teaspoons in every 20-ounce can of the two most popular brands) and a lot of caffeine. The active ingredient in the most popular cola drinks is phosphoric acid, which will dissolve a steel nail in four days. Phosphoric acid will also leach calcium from your bones, is a major contributor to the rising increase in osteoporosis (bone disease), and can do extensive damage to your teeth. One carbonated soda pop will counteract several days of taking calcium supplements by blocking calcium absorption, an essential nutritional building block. Studies show it takes 32 glasses of water with a pH of 9.0 to neutralize the acid from one 20-ounce soda pop, which registers 2.5 on the pH scale. Now, that's a lot of water to have to drink for one pop. The best thing to do is, don't drink pop.

Processed sugars (sucrose, a refined carbohydrate), as you might know, are extremely harmful to us and, if consumed regularly, can and will cause serious problems, including cancer. Two great books about sugar are *Sugar Blues* and *Licking the Sugar Habit*, by Nancy Appleton, Ph.D.

Processed sugars block the absorption of much-needed calcium, and deplete the vitamin B needed in our liver for detoxification. Too much sugar also robs us of needed oxygen in our cells and shuts down the immune system. Michael F. Jacobson, executive director of the Center for Science in the Public Interest and editor-in-chief of *Nutrition Action Health Letter* has said, "Concentrated sweets like white sugar and brown sugar, dehydrated cane sugar, raw sugar, turbinato sugar, maple sugar, maple syrup and other syrups, honey, and fructose, very much affect our blood sugars." These are all refined carbohydrates (carbs). Other refined carbohydrates include white flour, white rice, instant potatoes, and most packaged breakfast cereals. These products can affect blood sugar levels as quickly as concentrated sweets.

Michael F. Jacobson went on to say, "When sugar consistently accounts for 25% to 50% of caloric intake (the amount the majority of people of all ages are eating), the results are one or more serious health problems." High amounts of these sugars have been associated with an increase in triglycerides and higher levels of glucose and can be linked to cancer problems. We need to get off the "processed-sugar fix" and get it out of our lives. While doing this, it takes about three weeks or so for our bodies to stop craving sugar and for the mental cravings for sugar to pass. Cravings also subside when you give the body nutritional mineral supplements. Giving the body the proper amounts of minerals reduces these sugar cravings over time.

Eliminating processed sugar from your diet starts a natural mild detoxifying process. This is another time when nutritional supplements are important to take. If you have kids, it can be extremely hard to get them off sugar. One product that can help is Pro Vitamin Complete, which I use every day. It is a well-balanced liquid whole food supplement. There are also great natural sweeteners that will help you ease your way off sugar. I will talk about these products later. Considerable time and patience is required to cleanse the body of processed sugar, but it's well worth the effort.

Author and nutritionist Ann L. Gittleman has said, "Sugar destroys the ability of white blood cells to kill germs for up to five hours each time you eat it. It causes mineral imbalances which affects enzyme function, inhibits the actions of needed fatty acids, and leaves us vulnerable to invasion by allergens and micro-organisms."

Another highly used liquid sweetener is corn syrup. In 1971, high-fructose syrup was developed in Japan by Japanese food scientists. At this time, there was a big surplus of corn, which led to this new product discovery.

Corn syrup is formulated by using corn starch in several steps. The corn is cooked and separated from the husk and hull, then made into protein, starch, and oil. Finally, by using enzymes, it is converted from glucose into fructose. These are mixed together to create a high-fructose corn syrup sweetener that is roughly 55% fructose and 45% glucose, with other sugars added. Research shows this is the type of sweetener most drinks like pop and other products contain as a sweetener. These types of sweeteners are among the main causes of obesity in the United States today. Corn syrup is a cheap sweetener which helps hold the product price down.

This corn sweetener is six times sweeter than cane sugar and started replacing other sugars as its popularity and low price caught on in the market place. It is now used in 40% of all products that have sweeteners added. The average American consumes high amounts of corn syrup every day. Many consume up to 300 or more calories a day from vending machines, junk foods, sodas, sweetened fruit juices, cereals, cookies, snack bars, and many processed foods.

Between 1970 and 2000, the consumption of corn syrup has increased at least 10-fold.

This is a small part of a big puzzle when it comes to obesity, diabetes, and other problems caused by the consumption of high amounts of sugars in the American diet today. Adding corn syrup to your diet, along with a high caloric intake and lack of exercise, plays a big role in the exploding obesity problem we are seeing in our country today.

Avoid corn syrup and any kind of processed corn products. I avoid labels that say corn syrup, fructose, high fructose, cornmeal, cornstarch, corn oil, and so on. This sweetener is the most widely produced of all sweeteners on the market. One of the biggest changes you can make in your diet concerning sweeteners is to stop drinking sweetened drinks like soda pop, sweetened juices, and sweetened waters.

Don't be fooled with other so-called healthy drinks. Whatever they are called to attract attention, if it is sweetened, it will be filled with some type of sugar, usually a corn sweetener. Fructose, which is a natural sugar, can be just as dangerous as other sugars when you drink large amounts of sweet fluids. Eat your fruit, don't drink it. And if you have cancer, don't do either. I am saying this again, remember, *cancer loves sugar.* Artificial sweeteners are no better for you than natural sugar. They are actually worse.

Eating acid-forming foods, over time, can do extreme damage to the body, and is one of the most frequent causes of cancer, weak and brittle bones, dental decay, hyperactivity, and candida. These are just a few of the many problems you may encounter.

ARTIFICIAL CHEMICAL SWEETENERS

All products which have aspartame are extremely acid-forming and very harmful. Studies show aspartame may cause many serious medical problems, as well as cancer. It fits into the same category as these other artificial sweeteners. Diet sodas are the worst, as they are the highest in acid content. This acid can cause you to *gain* weight because it alters the body's blood chemistry and leads to a slower metabolic rate. This is a serious problem in our country right now. Get off all diet sodas, and artificial sweeteners, now.

Aspartame complaints are about 85% of the food complaints registered with the FDA. This chemical sweetener can have multiple neurotoxic, metabolic, allergenic, effect on a fetus, and carcinogenic effects on the body. Aspartame is a brain drug, meaning it stimulates your brain so you think the food you're eating or drinking tastes sweet. Research says this is why you crave carbohydrates when drinking it. It also breaks down into three different kinds of poison when heated to 86 degrees or higher. This could happen just by the cans sitting in your car on a hot day. These poisons are: aspartic acid 40%, phenylalanine 50%, and methanol 10%. Methanol toxicity mimics Multiple Sclerosis (MS) so patients are being misdiagnosed. Multiple sclerosis is not a death sentence but methanol toxicity is. Aspartame, and its brand of products that use it, also break down to form diketopiperazine (DKP) which has been proven to cause brain tumors in rats. With these findings out in the open you should never use aspartame, especially in hot beverages or cooked foods. An article by Nancy Markle, who spoke at the World Environmental Conference on Aspartame said, "Systemic lupus has become almost as rampant as MS, especially with diet soda consumers."

In 1991, the National Institute of Health listed 167 symptoms and reasons to avoid the use of aspartame because it caused such problems as brain tumors, birth defects, and multiple other diseases and disorders such as MS, ALS, blindness, migraines, and headaches, and is said to be deadly for diabetics. The list is long. These chemicals, after they break down in the body, attack the body's tissues and create formaldehyde. It then builds up in your tissues and remains forever. Research shows that the American Bottling Association did not want the FDA to approve aspartame, but the FDA went ahead with the approval anyway. Be sure to watch or buy a copy of the movie *Sweet Misery* and get off these artificial sweeteners now, no excuses!

Actor Michael J. Fox is a former diet soda spokesman, and is said to have been addicted to diet soda. Aspartame can precipitate Parkinson's disease, which he now has. Parkinson's affects a small patch of neurons in the brain called the *substantia nigra*. This patch of neurons produces the chemical dopamine, which the body uses to control movement. There is also evidence that the once strange disease that is now called Desert Storm Syndrome, and Burning Mouth Syndrome, from the 1991 war in the Persian Gulf, was partially caused from overheated diet pop containing aspartame, along with experimental vaccines and biological compounds the troops were exposed to. I know it seems strange that a little can of pop can do this amount of damage to us, but just remember what's in the can—poison. To understand different kinds of sugars, carbohydrates, and how to ease the sugar cravings better, check out these two sites: *www.livrite.com/sugar1.htm* and *askdrsears.com/html/4/to45000.asp.*

A recent study in Norway has shown aspartame destroys the brain, especially in the areas of learning, and this could account for the global epidemic of attention deficit disease.

Dr. John Olney, who was involved in the field of neuroscience, studied aspartame and found it causes lesions in the brains of mice. Neurosurgeon Russell Blaylock, M.D., wrote a book on this subject called, *Excitotoxins: The Taste That Kills*, and discussed Parkinson's disease at length in it. People, it's time to wake up and realize we are being poisoned and not told the truth!

When you drink soda, especially those containing artificial sweeteners, the deterioration rate of your body may be much faster and, over time, the effects of colas are devastating to your health. Even without drinking soda, your bodies produce acids and your stored minerals are used to stop the deterioration process caused by these acids, that is, if you still have any stored minerals left after drinking soda. In 1984, Dr. Harman, Ph.D., said, "Very few people reach their potential maximum life span. They die prematurely of a wide variety of diseases and the vast majority of these being free radical diseases." Free radicals are byproducts of the normal oxygen process within our bodies. These free radicals are unstable molecules inside us that attack stable molecular structures. These attacks, over time, cause damage to healthy tissues, organs, cell membranes, blood vessels, and DNA strands within the cells they attack. Free radical damage accelerates aging and aids the formation of disease. Antioxidants neutralize free radicals. The National Cancer Institute said, "free radical damage may lead to cancer."

Sucralose is a new sweetener on the market and currently, as of 2006, not much research has been done on its side effects. This product does contain chlorine. Some tests, however, have shown Sucralose may shrink the thymus gland, which is a foundation of the immune system, by as much as 40%. This artificial sweetener may also cause swelling of the liver and kidneys, calcification of the kidneys, and several other problems. It has been found to contain chloro-carbons which can cause organ, genetic and reproductive damage. You might want to look at the reference pages for more information on this and other sweeteners to avoid.

Sucralose is made from sugar but is derived from sucrose by a process that substitutes three atoms of chlorine for three hydrogen oxygen atom groups in the molecule of sucrose. Dr. Janet Hull says eating Sucralose is like ingesting tiny amounts of chlorinated pesticides.

GREAT ALTERNATIVE SWEETENERS

A well-known fact is that a diet excessively high in sugar (glucose) can be one of the major problems with the metabolic change of our system and the occurrence of malignant tumors. Cancer cells absorb and thrive on sugar as they multiply out of control. A diet high in any type of sugar will also significantly raise your chances of an onset of type II diabetes sometime in your midlife years.

A healthy and safe alternative sweetener is Thera Sweet™. It is made to be a safe and healthy alternative to regular and artificial sweeteners. Thera Sweet looks and tastes like sugar but doesn't have any of the bitter aftertastes. Xylitol is the main ingredient and comes from organic fruit sources. Tagatose is also added and it comes from yogurt and cheeses. Also, read about mannitol, sorbital, and xylitol sweeteners, from the websites in the reference pages.

An excellent natural herb sweetener you can buy at your local health food store is called "Stevia." This herb is native to Paraguay and the local Indians have used this herb for hundreds of years. Stevia is also safe for people with diabetes or hypoglycemia, over active kids and for people watching their weight. This is the main sweetener I use for teas and any other drinks I need to sweeten up.

Another great natural fruit sugar that can be used instead of processed sugars is Slim Sweet, and is made from the Lo Han fruit (a very sweet Chinese fruit). It is made from natural fruit concentrates with zero calories. Slim Sweet aids weight loss, promotes the burning of fat, supports healthy insulin levels, and is also safe for those with diabetes and hypoglycemia. This fruit sweetener is a great sweetener instead of refined sugars. Just think of the wonders that could happen to your body from its use.

If you are going to eat what we think of as regular sugar, or the white bleached stuff that we all know to be sugar, at least take a look at the new, all-natural (organic), sugars that are starting to make an appearance in our stores. Organic sugar has no pesticides or other toxic chemicals sprayed on their plants. One good website to take a look at a new sugar product is: *www.wholesomesweeteners.com*. This organic sugar is not a genetically modified organism (GMO) product and is therefore suitable for vegetarian, vegan, halal, (Muslim diet) gluten-free and plant-based diets. Further, it has not been bleached or colored, and the manufacturer doesn't use any animal byproducts in its production. I mention this form of sugar because new types of sugars are becoming more popular. If you're going to use sugar at all, it's better to use sugars as close to organic as possible. But to me, the only type of really organic sugars is the natural type we get when we eat organic foods. We only get the amount contained in that one particular piece of food.

Remember, if you have cancer, and want to fight it naturally, do not eat sugar. Sugar feeds cancer and cancer loves sugar. This means any type or any form of sugar—refined, concentrated, processed, natural, man-made or organic. This is very, very important.

NATURAL SUGARS WE DO NEED

Is it true our bodies need sugar? Yes it is! All the good sugar we do need comes from carbohydrates (carbs) such as vegetables, whole grains, and legumes. Refined carbs, as I mentioned earlier, can have serious consequences on our bodies and our health.

There are eight natural "saccharides" (natural sugars) we do need. In the last ten years, scientists have done extensive research on glyconutrients (glyco) and phytonutrients (phyto). This discovery is said to be one of the most important findings in years. These sugars have been known about for a long time, but are just now being studied closer. They are: glucose, galactose, fucose, mannose, N-acetyl-galactosamine, N-acetyl-glucosamine, N-acetyl-neuraminic acid and xylose.

These eight essential saccharides were also once abundant and common in the diets of our ancestors as they foraged for foods. Today, our foods have been stripped of these vital nutrients. This discovery is so important that four nobel prizes in medicine have been awarded because of it. Glyco means, "sweet nutrient." These eight sugars combine with proteins and fats in the body to create glycoforms, which coat the surface of every cell in the body. They act as cellular recognition molecules that communicate the messages our bodies need to function properly. Phyto means plant fats. Phytos are present in all fruits and vegetables and have been proven to modulate the effects of the immune system. Both glyco and phyto nutrients are needed to work together to enhance our immune system. *Harper's Biochemistry*, a textbook used by many medical schools in the United States was rewritten in 1996 to add an entire chapter listing these nutrients.

Today, our soils are depleted of necessary nutrients and our fruits and vegetables are not only sprayed with chemicals but are "green harvested." This means they are picked off the vine or pulled from the soil too early, when they are still developing and maturing on the vine, and before they have had a chance to ripen. Therefore, we get virtually none of the very important nutrients we need from these foods. When harvested and ripened correctly, scientists say the health benefits from these saccharides can be remarkable.

People can regain their ability to fight disease and infection and get their immune systems going again by eating the right kinds of foods such as these. Believe me, it works great. Read, *Sugars That Heal* by Emil Mondoa, M.D.

NOTES

<u>NOTES</u>

PART 5

FRUITS, FLAVONOIDS, ANTIOXIDANTS AND MORE

ELLAGIC ACID

All natural fruits are great for nutrition and for the immune system, but two fruits especially stand out for fighting cancer. These two fruits are red raspberries and pomegranates, and they are also very strong antioxidants. The fruits and seeds contain a large amount of ellagic acid. It has been clinically shown that ellagic acid causes apoptosis (cell death) in cancer cells. These fruits act as scavengers to bind to cancer-causing chemicals and make them inactive. They also prevent the binding of carcinogens to DNA, reducing the incidence of cancer. Scientists are now discovering that a vitamin and mineral deficiency can cause DNA cell damage over time. This can cause you to age prematurely, and could lead to cancer and other diseases such as Alzheimer's and Parkinson's, just to name a couple. Research in antioxidants in fruits and vegetables has also found antioxidants to help breast cancer, and cardiovascular disease, and depress tumor growth.

GSH

Glutathione (GSH), which is called the "master antioxidant," is made of three amino acids: glutamate, glycine, and cysteine. Cysteine is a form of an amino acid. No other nutrient is said to be more important for overall health. Russell Manuel, M.D., said, "Many people who suffer from chronic diseases have very low GSH levels in their bodies." Our cells produce GSH but as we get older GSH levels in our bodies drop, eventually making them more susceptible to disease. The average 65-year-old has at least 60% less GSH than when he or she were younger.

Twenty years of research at Montreal's McGill University Medical School has shown that raising our GSH levels is an effective way of combating cancer. Dr. Manuel, who started on this product when he was diagnosed with prostate cancer said, "I believe that my knowledge of GSH saved my life." He went on to say GSH helps many other health problems and diseases, along with clearing vision and improving cataracts.

GSH also helps to detoxify poisons, nicotine, and free-radicals in cigarette smoke, plays a big part in the body's defense against pollutants and ultraviolet radiation, and in the removal of heavy metals such as mercury, lead, and cadmium. Our bodies slow down in the production of GSH and the richest form of it is found in milk serum (whey) protein. This makes GSH suitable for lactose-intolerant people. This product can be found in your health food store.

There are many antioxidants that help us fight disease. Our immune system can become weak and less effective if we don't get the right nutrients. The proper liquid whole-food nutritional supplements contain the right amounts and ratios of the nutrients we need. This is why we need a superior liquid wholefood supplement that is highly absorbable allowing all the nutrients to interact.

ENZOGENOL AND PYCNOGONAL

Enzogenol and pycnogonal are two great flavonoids, which are a type of antioxidant. Antioxidants hunt down and neutralize free radicals that weaken our systems. When we consistently take antioxidants, cells regain their regeneration power and, once again, slow the aging process and accelerate healing the body. When free radicals go unchecked, they degrade collagen, reprogram DNA, and may cause more than 60 kinds of disease. Enzogenol and pycnogonal are found naturally in plant form. The kind I have found comes from pine tree bark extract from two different areas of the world, New Zealand and the United

States. These products can be up to 50 times more potent than vitamin E and 20 times more powerful than vitamin C. In addition, aging, inflammation, and improper functioning of the circulatory, nervous, and immune systems can result from free radical damage. There are many types of antioxidants in our foods but, when eating unhealthy diets we take in only very small amounts of these very important nutrients.

QUERCETIN

Another product, Quercetin, (kwer-se-ten) is a very important member of a large group of foods high in flavonoids. It is a plant pigment and an excellent antioxidant. Apples are one fruit high in flavonoids. Maybe it is true when "they" say, "An apple a day keeps the doctor away." Other fruits and vegetables high in flavonoids are raspberries (raspberries are also high in ellagic acid, which is known to kills cancer cells), black and green tea, red wine, red grapes, citrus fruits, cherries, and vegetables such as broccoli, leafy greens, and onions. These types of fruits and vegetables produce more healthy benefits than just flavonoids, so always try and eat fresh and organic. This is *very* important for your health.

Studies show Quercetin has anticancer effects, and helps prevent heart disease by reducing the oxidation of LDL (bad) cholesterol. Other studies done at the Mayo Clinic show flavonoids may also prevent prostate cancer by blocking the growth of prostate cancer cells, help with the inflammation of prostatitis, and help with lung cancer.

Dr. Nianzeng Xing Ph.D., a Mayo Clinic researcher, presented his study to the American Cancer Research Center in New Orleans, on March 26, 2001, during their 92nd annual meeting. His study showed Quercetin blocks the androgen hormone activity in human prostate cancer cell lines. He said, "By blocking the androgen activity, the growth of prostate cancer cells can be prevented or stopped."

Quercetin is a great natural nonhormonal product and treatment for prostate cancer. Prostate cancer claims 31,000 men, or about 11% of male cancer-related deaths in the United States each year. 200,000 men are diagnosed with prostate cancer each year in this country. Get busy and try to prevent prostate cancer or your number may come up next.

NONI JUICE

A nutritional drink called Noni juice, from the Noni fruit, is rich in essential fatty acids and promotes an alkaline environment for your body, which I talked about earlier. The scientific name for Noni is Morinda citrifolia. It grows well on sandy or rocky shores.

Noni is full of antioxidants critical in fighting off disease and free radicals that damage your cells. When free radical damage is under control, you are healthier and you will age more slowly.

This natural food supplement has been used by the Polynesian people for over 2,000 years to keep them healthy. Very important nutrients have been found in noni juice to help fight cancers, tumors, bacteria and much more. Dr. Steven Schechter, N.D., a nationally respected naturopathic physician said, "Noni fruit stimulates the immune system, regulating T-cell function and cellular regeneration of damaged cells."

The world's leading expert on Noni juice, biochemist Dr. Ralph Heinicke, identified an unknown compound in pineapple in 1972, while working with the Dole Pineapple Company. He gave it the name of "xeronine." He noted the importance xeronine has on our health, and set out to find other fruits that were rich in this nutrient. He discovered the Noni fruit contains enormous amounts of xeronine, 40 times more than pineapple, its closest competitor. Xeronine combines with protein in the body in order to allow it to function properly. It helps improve the natural ability for your body to heal itself. You may notice increased mental clarity and an increased attention span. Xeronine helps with the circulatory system, and assists with greater physical performance levels. Many people swear by this juice and testimonials show Noni to be a miracle juice, healing all kinds of problems.

Dr. Isabeela Abbott, a Professor at the University of Hawaii, says, "Use it for diabetes, high blood pressure, cancer, and many other illnesses." Recent studies of this wonder juice xeronine, shows that it stimulates the production of nitric oxide in the body.

Amazing new benefits of Nitric Oxide were discovered in 1998 by three researchers who won a Nobel Prize for medicine. It was found to be a signaling molecule involved in controlling blood circulation and regulating the brain and organs. Nitric oxide reduces tumor growth and stimulates the immune system. Noni has great health advantages just waiting for you, and contains over 150 health-promoting nutrients. This is truly an amazing juice. Don't pass up the chance to drink its healthy benefits for amazing results. Also check out Proxenol and Proxacine on your computer search engine. These are two excellent products that have been freeze dried using Noni.

People who are weak from cancer and chemo treatments, and have a hard time eating, can juice or have someone juice for them. Fresh vegetable juices from a juicer like beet root juice and carrot juice are excellent mixed together. Use about one fourth beet juice to three fourths carrot juice. Noni juice is also excellent, and is said to works wonders. These are great ways to start building some strength and energy. Drink the Noni juice separately from vegetable juice a couple hours apart because Noni comes from fruit. Noni is the only fruit juice I will drink when cancer is present and is said to be a great cancer fighter. Most other juices contain too much sugar. Remember, *cancer loves sugar*. Check out this Website: *www.cancer-prevention.net.* It will give you hope and has a lot of excellent information. It's quite lengthy. Set an hour aside so you can read and absorb the whole article and page-mark this website on your computer for later.

LAETRILE

In 1950, after many years of research, a biochemist named Ernst T. Krebs, found a new vitamin that he designated B17, and called it Laetrile. As years went by, thousands of people were convinced something had been found to control all cancers. More people still share that conviction today. It is said the pharmaceutical companies, unable to claim exclusive rights to the vitamin, launched a propaganda attack on Dr. Krebs' B17, saying it was not effective in controlling cancer. Dr. Krebs' evidence points to the fact that cancer is a simple deficiency disease of vitamin B17 which was removed from our highly refined western diet long ago. For generations, we used to crush the soft seeds of many fruits, all containing vital nutrients, and mix them in with jams and preserves.

Other research shows that a tribe of natives from the Himalayan region never contract cancer as long as they stick to their native diet, which is high in apricots. Dr. Krebs' B17 formula, made from apricot seeds, which contain cyanide, proved beyond a doubt that apricot pits are harmless when taken as he suggests. I have eaten apricot seeds that contain cyanide in large quantities and I am still here today. I ask you this, have you ever taken a B12 vitamin or a B complex vitamin? Or do you get a B12 shot every once in a while? If you do you might like to know B12 also contains quantities of cyanide, is still available in our stores today, and is safe to use.

Read the article mentioned in my reference pages called, "Laetrile: Another suppression story." It says if a person is going to try laetrile for cancer, it should be done *before* radiation and/or chemotherapy. When I eat apricot pits I sometimes eat almonds with them for a different taste. Almonds are also known to reduce inflammation in heart disease, cancer and other chronic degenerative diseases. Go to: *www.peopleagainstcancer.com* to find out more about it. This is a great site for people fighting cancer.

OTHER HEALING FRUITS

The next four fruits listed here all have excellent healing qualities. They are made into juices and some are also dried.

An exciting nutritional fruit comes from the Brazilian rain forest and is full of energy. It is the *acai* fruit (pronounced, ah-sigh-EE) and comes from the acai palm tree, which is called the "tree of life." Acai is a grape-size, deep-purple berry that grows on this species of palm tree in the jungle and contains the highest concentrated form of anthocyanins (a type of antioxidant) known to man. This little berry is known to be one of the most nutritious and powerful foods on earth. For the last ten years, acai has been studied by scientists around the world. It has been found to be rich in iron and fiber and helps to fight cholesterol and free radicals that cause disease. Acai has 33 times more anthocyanins than grapes, and is high in essential fatty acids. This fruit was mentioned on the Oprah TV show by a guest physician. The doctor pointed out that this fruit is the number one (out of ten) "super foods" for "age-defying beauty." Acai fruit is available in a liquid product and is one that I use quit often. Check for this in the reference pages.

Acai research from the Health Sciences Institute, July 2003 issue of *Nature's Perfect Food*, shows that plant pigments like anthocyanins can help prevent blood clots, improve blood circulation, relax blood vessels, and prevent artherosclerosis. Anthocyanins can also prevent cancer by blocking carcinogenesis on a molecular level and encourage tumor cell death. The benefits from this super liquid food keep piling up, and the news about its great benefits keep spreading.

The *Goji berry*, sometimes called wolf berry, is perhaps the most nutritious fruit on the planet. Goji berries date back hundreds of years in the Chinese dynasties. They contain 18 amino acids (six times higher than bee pollen), eight essential amino acids, and 21 trace minerals. These berries are rich in carotenoids, which have more beta-carotene than fresh carrots. They also have large amounts of vitamins C, B1, B2, B6, and E.

Dr. Earl Mindell, Ph.D., generally recognized as the world's leading nutrition authority says goji is the biggest discovery in nutrition in the last 40 years. He goes on to say, at long last the missing link has been discovered in the mountains of the Himalayas— a food so nutritionally dense that it is unmatched by any other substance on earth for its health-promoting powers. Goji is a treasure trove of four highly bioactive and unique polysaccharides (LBP1, 2, 3, 4) which are different and more active than anything science has seen before. Check it out at: *www.gojitools.com*.

Mangosteen is another super fruit you may have heard of by now. This fruit is made into a juice and is full of antioxidants to stimulate the immune system. It is antihistamine, antibacterial, antifungal and helps with antitumor activity. It also has anti-inflammatory properties and fights against cancer cells.

Capuacu, which is called the "taste of the gods" is another great fruit and health resource from the rain forest high in antioxidants, phytonutrients, and polyphenols. Capuacu has been proven to have an increased ability to fight disease and cancer. It also helps us to have a more youthful and healthier-looking skin and hair, lower cholesterol levels, and increases libido and stamina.

SOY CAN BE VERY BENEFICIAL

Soy, consumed on a regular basis, is extremely helpful when fighting disease as long as it is of the fermented variety like natto, amakaze, miso, and tempeh. These types of fermented soy stop the negative effects that regular, unfermented soy can have on your body. When using soy nutrients, you should only use fermented soy foods, not unfermented.

The nutrients that make up soy beans are anti-inflammatory, antibacterial, antiviral, antimutagenic, antiosteoporatic, and are an anticarcinogen. Soy has also been shown to reduce the incidence of different types of cancers and liver problems, lower cholestrol and more. Studies show taking a soy concentrate is much better than eating soy products because you cannot eat enough to be beneficial if the soy is not fermented.

Genistein and daidzein are two types of isoflavones in soy. Isoflavones are flavonoids that act as phytostrogons, which are useful in treating cancer. When fermented, they have been shown to slow skin cancer, leukemia, and lung, prostate, colon, and breast cancers.

Genistein and daidzein can be found in your health food store in capsule form. Tests also show these two nutrients, along with many other nutrients in fermented soy, can definitely help other diseases such as Parkinson's disease, muscular dystrophy, hepatitis, and the list goes on. One other very beneficial nutrient in soybeans is lecithin. I talk more about lecithin later.

Soy is difficult to digest when unfermented and may cause other problems. It has also been found that eating tofu products containing soy can be harmful, as soy in this form blocks the absorption of some important nutrients. However, when tofu is eaten with meat, these effects are reduced. Studies show a link between the brain's need for minerals and eating tofu to worsening dementia problems. Asian people have been sprouting and fermenting soy beans for hundreds of years. Eating fermented soy makes it easier for the body to digest and is much healthier.

Unfortunately, soybeans are, however, high in their own natural toxins (antinutrients). They contain goitrogens, which can slow thyroid function, and they have phytates which can stop the absorption of minerals such as calcium, magnesium, and zinc. Dr. Mercola's book, *Total Health Program* talks about soy products and is also an excellent book on nutrition, diets, and aging. Also, *The Whole Soy Story*, by Dr. Kaayla Daniel, is a great book on soy.

<u>NOTES</u>

NOTES

PART 6

---◆◆◆---

WHOLE FOODS FROM OUR LAND

GREEN FOOD CONCENTRATES

It is extremely important for you to keep your body healthy by eating the right kinds of foods, taking the right kinds and the right amounts of supplements, drinking the right amount of fresh water and exercising daily. Studies now show eating more vegetables like broccoli and other members of the same family, such as Brussels sprouts, bok choy, kale and turnips may stop the growth of breast cancer cells. Eating other vegetables such as sprouts, carrots, radishes, and beets is also healthy. Almost all green leafy vegetable are healthy. Buy a blender and see what you can come up with in different tastes with different vegetables and fruits. Blending vegetables is a great way to stay healthy and is fun to do. Get your kids involved while they're young. Let them help with their own healthy vegetable drink. They will love it.

Remember, taking too many, or the wrong kinds of nutrients may also be bad for your body. We need natural nutrients, not the man-made ones that come in little hard pills that your body has a hard time dissolving. You need a natural, blended combination of unrefined food to provide you with all the nutrients you need. That's why I think a whole-food liquid supplement works the best, especially for people on the go. Nutritional products do work and are powerful. If we take too many of one kind, especially oil based vitamins, it can offset the balance of nutrients, and you may overdose, making you feel sick and sluggish.

Nutritional supplements in capsule or liquid rather than hard pills can be good too, but make sure you find a company that makes a good supplement. Ask questions at your local health food store regarding good products. In this book, I also talk about Pro Vitamin Complete, which is a liquid whole-food supplement I think is one of the superior liquid products on the market.

Now that we're talking about whole foods I should mention powdered green food concentrates. There are many different types and brand names of green foods that are extremely important for us and have just about everything a body needs for great health.

Two of the most important types of greens we can eat are chlorella and spirulina. These two superfoods are also called "micro-algae" since they are a type of algae. When used together, they contain amazing amounts of almost everything we need for excellent health. Many consider them to be a whole food.

Some green formulas contain chlorella, which is rich in chlorophyll, protein, vitamins, minerals, and is one of the richest sources of nutrients on the planet. Chlorella belongs to the eukaryotic family of algae which means "visible nuclei." It is a small single-celled plant that grows in fresh water. Chlorella means "small green leaf."

Spirulina is a blue-green algae and may be among the oldest plant forms on earth. It is rich in phytonutrients, which significantly boost the immune system. It also has carotenoid antioxidants, which reduce the risk of cancer and help with detoxifying the body. This great food is known to go way back to the days of the Aztecs in Mexico, over five centuries ago.

Many people consider beef or other meats to be the number one source of protein, but this is incorrect. Spirulina offers us 20 times more protein than beef. It is a vegetable protein containing high amounts of beta carotene, vitamin B-12, iron, trace minerals, and the essential fatty acid gamma-linolenic acid (GLA). Don't forget, unless you eat "free- range" beef, you are also getting plenty of chemicals and hormones that have been added to the beef, passing these cancer-causing agents on to you and now becoming your problem. These two superfoods spirulina and chlorella have no toxins and are rich in phytonutrients such as phycocyanin, polysaccharides, and sulfo-lipids. Phytonutrients enhance the immune system and help cut the risk of cancer and autoimmune diseases.

Chlorella is a superhealthy food that helps detoxify the body of heavy metals that have accumulated over a lifetime. Even small amounts of this plant can help the body repair DNA and give you much more needed energy. Chlorella and spirulina should definitely become part of your diet. One thing I enjoy eating as a supersnack, usually between meals, is a spirulina ball. The spirulina, along with other healthy ingredients, is rolled up into a silve-dollar-size ball, then covered with crushed almonds. This is a very healthy and tasty snack. I buy these in a 40- or 70-count tub and eat a couple a day. I definitely don't like to run out of these snacks. They will get you by until your next healthy meal is ready. I talk about the snacks I ate when I had cancer, and still eat today, later in the book.

Chlorella can also help you in the dentist's chair while having cavities filled or extracted by protecting you from the toxic effects of mercury fillings, also called 'silver fillings' (amalgam). In 1992, California governor Pete Wilson paved the way for looking into these types of fillings, hoping to ban the use of mercury in dental restoration. This brought thousands of dentists, around the country, to call for such a ban. California is also the first state to pass legislation on chlorella, which helps escort mercury out of your body before it can do damage and is said to be a mercury magnet. Research has shown that this superfood can also be used by the body to aid in the breakdown of toxins such as DDT, PCB, cadmium, and lead. Having chlorella in your stomach, when you are swallowing pieces of mercury as in the dentist's chair, for instance, can be beneficial. I am in the process of having my mercury fillings removed and replaced with white (composite) fillings or gold or white crowns, because of the dangers of disease from mercury.

Mercury is a known poison and one of the most toxic of all elements. It can travel to all parts of the body through the blood and collect in your tissues. Depending on where it collects in the body, it can do damage in several ways by causing depression, kidney disease, Alzheimer's, cancer, and more. Sweden and Germany have strict laws in place to significantly curb the use of mercury fillings, and Canada is said to follow suit soon.

The World Health Organization shows studies that one single amalgam filling can release 3 to 17 micrograms of toxic mercury per day into your body. This makes dental fillings a major problem for mercury exposure. But little is being done. Most dentists are still saying these types of fillings are safe and continue this practice although mercury is more toxic than arsenic. Go to: *www.PeopleAgainstCancer.com.*

The biological holistic dentistry approach is catching on in the United States with dentists concerned about toxic metals such as mercury, and some are quickly adapting new ideas in this field for their patients. Mercury is extremely bad for the body and your immune system. In the early 1900's, the National Association of Dental Surgeons wanted to do away with mercury amalgam. The cheapness of the product, however, kept it in use and it was soon said to be safe. Fortunately, we now know the truth.

If you want a great natural appetite suppressant, want to reduce your cravings and be healthier, try eating a supergreen formula. There are many causes of sugar cravings such as mineral deficiencies, and yeast overgrowth (candida). Because of the protein chlorella and spirulina contain, they will help fill you up and take your cravings away for a short period while you are absorbing the nutrients. If you have a nervous system disorder, a good green formula with a combination of these two super foods can repair nerve tissues over time.

If you have cancer, you definitely need to be taking these two superfoods for their cancer-preventing and cancer-reversing properties. Spirulina is also rich in pyycocyanin and is the highest plant source of GLA which inhibits cancerous cell division. I could go on and on about the great benefits of these two superfoods but you should check these out for yourself. Check the reference pages and websites.

ORGANIC FOOD AND WHOLE-FOOD SUPPLEMENTS

Let's take a look at "natural whole (organic) food." Organic food is intended to be eaten in its pure form. These whole foods are foods that have been produced by nature and are kept in their natural organic state until eaten. These are natural foods that *have not* been sprayed, preserved, or altered in any way. This is the way we need to be eating our food. The lack of these types of foods in our diet will contribute to health problems and a run-down immune system if not corrected.

Whole foods are good old everyday fruits, vegetables, meats, and grains, of which some of us eat very little since fast foods and processed foods have come along. Organic foods are not processed, refined, or genetically altered (engineered) foods. Organic foods have not been grown with chemical fertilizers, sprayed with toxic chemicals, or injected with chemicals. An organic farmer must adhere to strict standards and undergo regular inspections to ensure that he meets all standards for organic growing. There now seems to be a problem with the real meaning of *organic, natural, grass-fed,* and *free range.* These are some of the words the U.S. Department of Agriculture (USDA) is using to help define, or redefine, the word *organic,* and at this point, consumers are naturally confused about the definitions of these new words popping up in the marketplace.

The word *natural* doesn't mean the meat is automatically free of toxic chemicals, hormones and antibiotics anymore. What it does mean is that animals raised "naturally" are still subject to reduced doses of toxic chemicals, which are passed on to us. It does not mean they are let out of their cages or pens to roam freely.

The word *grass-fed* is used for beef, and *free-range* is used for poultry. These animals are said not to be confined to cages or indoors but may still be fed chemical toxins in the feed they eat. "Organically" raised animals must meet all stringent health conditions and must be given only organic grain as approved by a USDA-approved certifier.

Be careful when buying seafood. The USDA does not have standards for organic fish as of April, 2006. Companies are free to make claims as long as they don't claim them to be organic. Our oceans are being overloaded with toxic waste and fish can have heavy metals and toxins in them such as mercury and PCBs. Be careful when purchasing fish. PCBs are toxic chemicals know as polychlorinated biphenyls. They are man made and are not natural. To read more go to: *http://dep.state.ct.us/wst/pcb/pcbindex.htm* or see my section on chemicals in this book.

According to *Energy Times*, April 2006, sales of organic food and drinks reached $15 billion in 2004, and are estimated to double by 2009, with organic sales having increased 17% to 21% each year since 1997 in the U.S. marketplace. Remember, if you're a little confused when you go to the store and start to see these new labels while you're shopping, just ask your grocer if it's truly organic. If not, "Just say no." Make sure to look for foods that say "100% organic." If it just says "organic" on the label, it may not be 100% organic.

If you do not eat organic foods and do not eat an abundance of fruits, vegetables and protein, your body desperately needs a whole-food liquid supplement. I now eat the proper foods but I also take Pro Vitamin Complete™ every day. This is an excellent product for our nutritional needs. In our fast-paced world, very few of us get balanced food supplements in the diets we eat. Pro Vitamin Complete has 178 superfood ingredients for a great nutritional liquid product. Some of us pop a few vitamins here and there but these usually are not enough for our bodies' needs.

Pro Vitamin Complete contains:
13 natural vitamins
23 whole food greens
 4 essential fatty acids
 7 plant enzymes, concentrate blend
63 proprietary ionic trace minerals from organic sea vegetation
 6 multifibers
28 fruit and vegetable phytonutrients
18 protein amino acid liquids
a proprietary super herbal complex
ellagic acid from pomegranate and red raspberry extracts

This is a complete wholefood liquid nutritional supplement. Very few other products I have mentioned come close to all the nutritional components in this great tasting, easily absorbed supplement that kids and parents love because it taste great. It is one that you'll want to keep around to maintain the health of your whole family. See my website in the rear of this book for this product.

Dr. Richard Wiseman, M.D., had this to say about Pro Vitamin Complete. "Over the last 33 years I have practiced pediatrics, obstetrics, emergency medicine, and family medicine. In all my years, I have never encountered a formula that was designed for children, adults, and the elderly that provided "complete" nutrition for every part of the human anatomy. I recommend this to all my patients."

One way to make sure we get all of our nutrients when healthy foods are not available, is by taking a whole-food supplement that has all the nutrients we need every day. Why is this so important? These are the nutrients that keep us alive. Even some organic foods today have fewer of these life-giving nutrients than ever before because of the soil they are grown in. Pro Vitamin Complete has ionic minerals, which I believe is a very important aspect of this product. As I mentioned, in the minerals section of this book, ionic minerals, compared to colloidal minerals, come straight to us from the plant. Ionic minerals are the smallest form of minerals there is, and are more readily available for the body to use.

We are surrounded with new types of processed foods that our bodies don't know what to do with after we eat them. Our foods are sprayed, injected, mixed, overcooked, processed, modified, dyed, and canned with deadly toxins and growth hormones of many kinds. We are also filling our bodies with dead foods that have no nutritional value and foods that are oversweetened, oversalted, and contain all kinds of artificial chemical diet sweeteners. Where are we headed with all of this? Down the road to disease!

If you think you're a person who would have a hard time changing your nutritional habits, you're not alone. Many people don't know where to start. One easy way to start is with a whole-food liquid supplement that has all the nutrients in one bottle, is easy to swallow, tastes great, and one that kids love instead of choking on hard vitamin pills or taking nothing at all. Not only are pills hard to swallow, but hard vitamin pills are said not to absorb as easily. This product definitely does not have the dreaded vitamin aftertaste.

People shouldn't feel frustrated when trying to find nutritional products and supplements. You should find one that the whole family agrees on and everyone will like because of taste, and which can be easily swallowed. Start out slowly. Find what your family's needs are, and go from there. Make it a lifestyle change and it will make a *big* difference in the long run for your family. Read and educate yourself and, as you become more interested, you will naturally follow a better health plan for the whole family. Don't pick the road to disease. Please see my personal websites on page 209 for this ProVitamin product.

If you keep ignoring your health, your health will eventually ignore you and your body will start to form some type of disease. Dr. William Albrech, of the University of Missouri, in talking about our soil depletion said, "The problem is rapidly reaching the size of catastrophe and, if carried much further, could mean national suicide. Soil health is that important."

Our vegetables should contain the majority of our micronutrients (vitamins, minerals, fiber, phytochemicals).Vegetables rich in color indicate a higher nutritional value. Dark greens, reds, yellows, and purples are high in nutrients. Organic vegetables are just a little higher in price, but are also higher in nutrients and have no toxins. Organic farms do not use chemical fertilizers, pesticides, or herbicides. If you're in a place where organic vegetables are impossible to find, soak your vegetables and fruits in vinegar for 10 to 15 minutes and then wash thoroughly before cutting. Soaking vegetables and fruits in vinegar will help to remove toxins (sprays) from your food.

<u>NOTES</u>

<u>NOTES</u>

PART 7

SUPER FOODS FROM THE SEA

SEA VEGETATION

"Sea vegetation," also called "seaweed" or "sea plants", has been used as a food, as a nutritional supplement, and as a wrap for skin care for thousands of years, as far back as 2700 BC. Sea vegetation provides hundreds of organic compounds, is toxin free, and does not absorb toxic chemicals as it grows. It is one of the Earth's healthiest forms of food. Sea vegetation contains a full spectrum of organic nutrients and compounds that bind to toxins, which are then flushed out of the body. Some of the earth's greatest treasures are beneath our oceans. Research has proven that some of the richest sources of minerals come from these waters. As our soils become more and more depleted from growing our crops, we need to look more toward our oceans for nutrients to protect ourselves from all diseases. Seaweed offers nutrients almost impossible to find from our soils and is a balanced form of nutrition essential to help live a healthy life. The product of seaweed I use is called Sea Vegg™; it is an ocean blend of 12 nutritionally dense species of sea plants. Go to: *www.tryseavegg.com* to find out more about this great product.

MODIFILAN

The brown seaweed, fucoidan (Laminaria japonica) an extract from the "center core" of the brown seaweed plant, is excellent for fighting cancer, and contains the life-essential properties of organic iodine, alginates, fuocoidan and laminarin. Organic iodine regulates our metabolism for better overall health. Alginate is a natural absorbent of radioactive elements, heavy metals, and free radicals. And excellent brand name for fucoidan is Modifilan. It is the one I use along with the product Sea Vegg, which has many types of seaweed products in one tablet. These two products are excellent and are all natural and organic.

The nutritional powers of seaweed have been known for thousands of years but the scientific health benefits have been established only recently. One of the healthy aspects of Modifilan is that this seaweed product is very high in polysaccharides. Ongoing research shows that fucoidan has the ability to induce cell death among cancer cells such as stomach, colon, and leukemia cancer. It has also contributed to the amazingly low breast cancer rates that have been reported in Japan.

Research shows Fuocoidan kills cancer cells, and laminarin-polysaccharide is helpful in the prevention of cardiovascular disease.

Fuocoidan exhibits about 30% of the anticoagulant activity of heparin. Fuocoidan is quite different from plain, dried seaweed. It is an extract of the very rich core of the seaweed plant. It takes up to forty pounds of raw seaweed to make one pound of fuocoidan. It's an amazing seaweed byproduct and is widely used in Japan for all kinds of health problems and diseases. It is used to lower cholesterol levels, high blood sugar, is an antiviral and anticancer agent, aids in digestion and elimination, increases energy, and strengthens the immune system. It has also been used to detoxify heavy metals and radioactive elements in the body, to slow or stop tumor cells, and to aide in poor thyroid function, and cardiovascular diseases.

Fucoidan is an excellent food supplement and is best taken on an empty stomach, such as in the morning, and will not cause nausea but gives a feeling of well-being. A big 40% of this super seaweed is alginates

(*Algal polysaccharides*). This not only helps to remove toxins in the food we eat, but also with toxins like radiation in the air and on the ground from nuclear plant fallout, microwaves, high voltage power lines, computers, and televisions. These are only a few, but they do contribute to free radicals in our bodies that cause many kinds of problems such as aging, leukemia, birth defects, and cancers.

The human body is bathed in a saline solution almost the same as the ocean. Seaweed fits right in with the body's healing powers. If you currently have cancer, I would definitely put this on your list, as I did. It is time to take a really hard look at what our environment is doing to our bodies and then we must do something about it, today.

SEA SALT

Our bodies are oceans of water and when we are eating properly, compare closely to ocean water. The plasma in our blood, our lymphatic circulatory system and the water around our cells are bathed in our body's water constantly. These bodily fluids are vital to our existence and have a definite role in the functions of our bodies' performance.

The regular white, refined, table salt we have grown up with is unnatural by the way it is processed. Most of the essential trace minerals and other nutrients have been removed through the refining process, leaving mostly sodium chloride. It is important that we use natural sea salt, which contains the correct percentage of magnesium salts (between .75 to 1.5%). This puts us in harmony with the body's cellular fluids. Japanese women have a very low incidence of breast cancer compared to Americans. And Japanese men have a lower incidence of prostate cancer than American men because of iodine. The Japanese eat about 100 times more iodine because of their diet rich in seaweed. Iodine plays a big part in killing cancer cells, so make sure you get enough in your diet.

Salt is important in our diets as long as it is the correct type of salt and not refined, like the iodized salt most of us use. Nature puts 84 essential trace minerals in sea salt to help guard us from health problems. When salt is washed, refined, or kiln-dried, these important minerals are remove—something we really don't think about when eating table salt. Studies show a diet without salt can damage the valves of the heart, cause sexual and glandular problems (such as goiters), and reduce the effectiveness of our immune system. Our bodies run on salt. Without it we would run out of electrolytes and our energy levels would severely drop. Salt is also an energizer and helps rebuild our cells. Because sea salt contains such an abundance of minerals, it helps with all types of diseases and problems. It also helps with enlarged prostates, to dissolve kidney stones, and can help arrest some forms of cancer.

Magnesium is one of the major components in sea salt and one of the major minerals needed to keep us healthy. In the proper amounts, it can help cure serious diseases, and improve enlarged prostates, help to dissolve kidney stones, and help with some forms of cancer. Magnesium salts make our bodies run smoothly, and without it we would suffer serious consequences. It stimulates our white blood cells and, when used on wounds or with other diseases, it accelerates the healing process. It also helps with many other problems such as psoriasis, eczema, acne, and herpes.

When our magnesium intake is low we may have a craving for salt. When we try to replace the salt by eating refined table salt, this can sometimes lead to an over-consumption of salt. Sea salt contains minerals our body needs and can replace needed minerals without the harmful effects we would get from regular table salt. Researchers say that refined table salt is completely unnatural and is stripped of all natural nutrients by the way it is refined. This can be dangerous to our health.

Dr. Esteban Genao, a pediatrician in Florida, has said, "Celtic Sea Salt has the ability to keep all bodily fluids in a balanced state. When a body exists in this state of equilibrium, the immune system will be strong, the metabolism will be healthy and our organs will function easily. Celtic Sea Salt benefits the whole body."

<u>NOTES</u>

NOTES

PART 8

———◆———

SUPER HERBS

PAW PAW HERB

The Paw Paw herb, which comes from the common Paw Paw tree that grows in the midwestern states, has been studied for years by Dr. Jerry McLaughlin.

Paw Paw has now been confirmed to be a beneficial help in the fight against all types of cancer, even brain, breast, prostate, and colon cancer. Studies show that in patients taking the Paw Paw herb, it is typical to see a significant reduction in the size of tumors and antigen levels within six to eight weeks.

The Paw Paw tree has a European cousin called gaviola, but it is said to be not as potent as Paw Paw. People using Paw Paw in the United States are finding that its benefits are boosted when it is taken with digestive enzymes (Protease enzymes) and a good quality Noni juice.

You will also see an increase in energy level because your healthy cells no longer have to compete with the cancer cells for energy. In addition, this herb has been found to help shingles, acne, lice, and cold sores, just to name a few other helpful benefits.

Dr. McLaughlin discovered that Paw Paw contains a group of plant chemicals called annonaceous acetogenins (known as fatty acids) and has over 50 types of these fatty acids. According to Dr. McLaughlin, these acetogenins can kill diseased cells that are resistant to chemotherapy drugs and is up to 300 times more potent than the drug Taxol, without causing weight loss. This is an amazing herb. I'm taking it myself. Pregnant women should not use this product at all. Always consult your doctor first. People without cancer should not use it long-term. People who have Parkinson's disease should not take this unless alkaloid-free preparations are made and used.

Studies show Paw Paw had no toxic effects when used with laboratory animals. Men with prostate cancer showed evidence of tumor reduction and their PSA numbers decreased. Paw Paw has been used with many different types of tumors with significant reductions in size, along with reduction in tumor antigen levels. Very few unwanted effects have been found when using Paw Paw. This is one of the main herbs I have relied on throughout my fight with cancer. I am still here, I am not dead, and I have no side effects from this herb at all. After using this herb, I have noticed I have more energy and I fight off colds and flu much more easily.

BLACK SALVE

Black Salve which dates back a couple of hundred years is another great herbal healer from the American Indians, and is still known today as an excellent healer. I found that two preparations are available. One type is oral and the other is a salve. It can be used internally and externally with great results in all areas of healing. It is called Black Salve because of the herbs it is made from. When the herbs are combined they turn black. Case histories have revealed that formulating the proper proportions of the various herbs can result in a wide variety of healing. This combination of herbs has not only been used as a salve, but also for internal malignancies in the liver, kidneys, colon, prostate, female sex organs, breast, lung and throat areas, and against a variety of viruses, fungi, and bacteria. The salve works for sun skin damage, warts, moles and other skin problems. I definitely recommend looking into this one.

CAYENNE PEPPER

Cayenne pepper is a member of the fruit family, coming from the fruit of the red pepper plant. "Cayenne" is a Greek word meaning "to bite" and targets the digestive and circulatory systems. Capsaicin, found in cayenne pepper, is what makes it hot. It is one of nature's most powerful stimulants and can make prostate cancer cells kill themselves.

Cayenne detoxifies and regulates blood pressure, strengthens the pulse, helps lower cholesterol, thins the blood (dissolves clots), cleanses the circulatory system, helps to heal ulcers, stops hemorrhaging, speeds healing and supports the viscera and internal rhythm of the glandular, circulatory, lymphatic, and digestive systems. Cayenne pepper restores normal functions in the body and is a superb medicine to keep our systems working the way they should. Cayenne stimulates every system and every cell of the body. It helps arteries, veins, and capillaries by revving up the circulatory system and restoring elasticity by feeding the cell structure with healthy blood and nutrients. It also helps the body's fibrinolytic system, which helps prevent blood clots from forming, and dissolves other clots already formed.

Dr. Soren Lehmann of the Cedars-Sinai Medical Center and the University of California Los Angeles School of Medicine, said "Capsaicin had a profound antiproliferative effect on human prostate cancer cells in culture."

Cayenne capsaicin stops the NF-kappa beta activity that leads to apoptosis (cell death) in many types of cancers. Cancer, like many diseases, can be caused by a lack of proper circulation, which may be sluggish circulation without the proper oxygen and nutrients. Capsaicin, one of the potent chemicals in cayenne pepper, helps protect DNA and cells from free-radical damage and increases blood flow to all parts of the body, including cancer sites. It also helps with tonsillitis, sore throats, scarlet fever, and diphtheria. The list is long of the benefits of this great fruit (herb). Cayenne pepper is excellent for the body. It wakes the body up, gives it a kick in the butt, and makes it run smoothly.

Researchers at two medical institutions discovered that cayenne prevents the liver from turning the polyaromatic hydrocarbons in smoked and broiled meat, and the afatoxins in peanut butter into carcinogens.

MAITAKE, REISHI, AND SHIITAKE

Highly respected in Japanese herbal medicine is the maitake mushroom. Pronounced (myTAHkay), it is considered an excellent herb that will strengthen glands and organs. Anticancer research shows that maitake works in killing prostate cancer cells, causing apoptosis (cell death) activity in cancerous cells and works well with patients having various other advanced cancers being threatened by chemo. Maitake was also found almost as effective when used by itself without chemotherapy. A good mixture I use is maitake, reishi, and shiitake mushrooms, since all three have properties that fight cancer.

AMAZING GARLIC

Garlic is a wonder food in a lot of ways. As early as 3000 BC, Chinese scholars were using garlic for many diseases. In 1500 BC, Egyptian physicians were using garlic for all kinds of complications. In World War I and World War II soldiers used garlic to treat wounds. Garlic has been used in helping to prevent disease and colds, mostly because of its antioxidant ability, effectiveness as a natural antibiotic, and the organic compounds found in it. But it can cause indigestion and bad breath for some people. If this happens to you, there are different strengths and kinds of garlic you can take.

Research has found that garlic's natural antibiotics kill the bacteria that cause disease. Garlic is a natural immune booster and when used daily, helps to slow the aging process. Garlic helps with cardiovascular problems, lowers bad cholesterol (LDL), lowers blood pressure, raises good cholesterol (HDL), helps with atherosclerosis, cuts the risk of heart attacks, and reduces the painful symptoms of sickle cell anemia. Recent studies show evidence of significant reduction in oxidative damage from smoking, and lowering the risks of colon, prostate, and stomach cancer. Garlic also protects against viral, bacterial, and yeast infections, allergies, candida, diabetes, aging, and reduced memory and brain functions. Garlic helps prevent blood vessel blockage by inhibiting the tendency of the blood cells to stick together and form clots. I use this in a circulatory flush I will mention later.

Research has also found the garlic you use does not have to be fresh, and is even better when it is given the chance to age, in its natural state, up to 18 to 24 months. The strong smell of garlic is not important for its health benefits to be noticed. Garlic has also been known as an antistress herb and fights DNA damage from free radicals damaging our cells. Aged garlic, in a highly concentrated form, has a sulfur compound called S-allylmerapto-cysteine (SAMC), which is said to have valuable anticancer properties especially effective in prostate cancer.

TURMERIC

Turmeric, also called curcumin, is another great herb for fighting cancer. Turmeric has mainly been used in Asian cooking for thousands of years. According to scientists at the University of Chicago, turmeric inhibits a cancer-provoking bacteria associated with colon and gastric cancer. Tests are ongoing for turmeric's anti-inflammatory and anticarcinogen properties.

Tests in Germany in 2003 found turmeric to be more potent than garlic, devil's claw and salmon oil for antioxidant activity. It is said that several other studies show turmeric slows the development and growth of a number of different types of cancer cells. A good turmeric web site that will explain more on this is: *www.psa-rising.com/eatingwell/turmeric.htm*.

OTHER GREAT HERBS

A few other herbs, teas, syrups, tonics, elixirs, and salves for cancer and other diseases are: Pau D'Arco, which is known around the world for its cancer-fighting properties. *Salvia lyrata*, also called the cancer weed, and lyre leaf lage. Chinese white tea is great for a strong immune system and you may have heard of green tea, already. Laboratory studies show the L-theanine found in green tea may help with the destruction of cancer cells. California yew and chaparral teas are also great cancer fighters. Trifolium (red clover) and scrophularia herb formulas are shown to work in fighting cancer. Carctol, a mixture of eight herbs, is known in Great Britain and India as a completely safe herbal supplement and has up to a 40% success rate with terminal cancer patients.

There is a variety of some 2.5 million herbs categorized as cytotoxic (toxic to cancer cells). These herbs date back some 5,000 years. At least 3,000 of these herbs have anti-cancer properties of some kind. The way these herbs help with disease is different for each herb. There is probably a bigger variety of cytotoxic herbs than there are chemotherapeutic drugs.

"The difference between drugs and herbal remedies is that, even though some drugs are derived from herbs, the majority of drugs are synthetic and work against the body, while herbs work in concert with the body to balance and allow true healing to take place." (www.1cure4cancer.com).

For a list of some of the Chinese herbs used for cancer go to: *www.herbsforcancer.com/herbs.html.*

<u>NOTES</u>

NOTES

PART 9

HERBAL TEAS
AND HEALTHY COFFEE

ESSIAC TEA

For every illness I believe there is an herb, or combination of herbs, that will help overcome it. One of these that should not be forgotten is Essiac Tea, which has a mixture of very important herbs for fighting cancer. In 1959, Charles Brusch, M.D., said "Essiac Tea, has merit in the treatment of cancer."

In 1922, Rena Caisse, who was a nurse at Sisters of Providence Hospital in northern Canada, opened a clinic and treated her patients with Essiac Tea. Initially, she healed herself of breast cancer, through the help of an Indian living in the area who showed her what herbs to collect and made a tea from these herbs. Being excited about her cure, she went on to help others, soon gained other doctors' support, and from 1935 to 1941 treated thousands of patients.

In 1977, when she was 89, she signed her recipe over to a company in Ontario, Canada. She is remembered for her contribution in helping so many people and not charging one penny for her services. Make sure to read her story about the mixture of these combined healing herbs. Look at the reference pages for *Essiac Tea, Rena Caisse's Story*, or look on your computer search engine. Also, an article in the issue of *Wildfire*, Vol. 6 No.1 mentions, "Ted Kennedy's son was treated with Essiac Tea at Brusch Medical Centre in Massachusetts by Dr. Charles Brusch." Dr. Brusch had cancer of the lower bowel which completely disappeared after Essiac Tea treatments. This tea contains the powerful herbs of the Burdock root, sheep sorrel, slippery elm bark, and Turkish rhubarb. Both Essiac and Flor-Essence (below) are powerful detoxifiers for the body. These herbs work to remove toxins, free radicals and chemical waste from our organs and blood stream. Essiac and Flor-Essence also cleanse the intestinal track and remove sluggish waste to improve digestion for great health and energy.

FLOR-ESSENCE

Another purification (detox) tea is called Flor-Essence. It is a liquid herbal tea which started with the Essiac Tea recipe. This great product contains the herbs in Essiac Tea, plus three more herbs: watercress, blessed thistle, and red clover blossom. This tea was entrusted to President Kennedy's personal physician, Dr. Charles Brusch, who was a partner in research and co-owner with Rena Caisse in perfecting this formula at their Massachusetts clinic. Here, they used this formula to help thousands of people. Flor-Essence liquid gently flushes the toxins from the kidneys, liver, lungs, colon, bloodstream, and the deepest cells in the body. This is the only product like this on the market that has Elaine Alexander's (herbalist) signature on the bottle to show its authenticity and to verify that it contains the same real herbs used back in 1922.

Environmental toxins and food chemicals of hundreds of different kinds can build up in our bodies and cause long-lasting problems, disease, and even death. We need to know how to get rid of these poisons so our bodies can be restored to a healthy balance. Toxins can remain in our bodies for minutes or for a lifetime, depending on the types we absorb or breathe in.

You need to detoxify your body to restore it to its natural balance and overall health. Chemical toxins are flushed mostly from the organs through the skin, liver, and kidneys, and finally flushed out of the body. Make sure you drink plenty of water during any flushing process.

Herbs in Essiac Tea and Flor-Essence are good products to start with to detoxify the body. Also, be sure to exercise. Exercise raises your metabolism and helps in the detoxification process. There is a special exercise that works well when detoxifying called "rebounding," which I mentioned previously. I have used both of these products myself. I used Essiac Tea to start with, which can be made stronger if needed, or to preference. It usually can be found in a box, as loose herbs. These herbs need to be boiled. Sometimes the tea can be found in liquid form. Once a year I use Flor-Essence tea, after a 12-week regimen with Essiac, as a follow-up or continuation. Flor-Essence comes in liquid form ready to drink. A good website on this is at: *www.florahealth.com*.

KOMBUCHA TEA

Another great immune booster is Kombucha Tea, pronounced (Com-boo-cha). Kombucha Tea has been called the "miracle cure-all" for hundreds, if not thousands, of years. It was made at home long ago as the "secret formula" for rulers, kings, and presidents, and now, for anyone wanting to use it. It is a powerful health drink that has been the answer to many health problems. It will boost your ability to fight sickness and disease and bring balance back to your metabolism and organs. It can still be made at home, or you can buy it from your health food store. I found out that if you buy it in your health food store, always buy the liquid form. It is much more potent and fresh in this form. I have found when I make this product at home it is *very* fresh and seems to work better, with more of a punch.

Kombucha Tea has been around long enough that chemists, researchers, medical professionals, and even the FDA have been interested in it. Kombucha, as it ferments, forms a yeast culture. This yeast culture, referred to as a mushroom, is said to be the oldest food and medicine of mankind. Kombucha was known during the Chin Dynasty around 221 B.C. and was used as an elixir for immortality. Eventually this knowledge spread throughout the world and became cherished by the Romans, Japanese, Koreans, Russians and other cultures. In 1983, Ronald Reagan used Kombucha Tea for cancer. This culture is made of various yeasts, which are self-produced as the mushroom grows and the tea ferments.

The kombucha culture is a form of membrane and is a symbiosis of yeast cells and bacteria such as *Bacterium xylinum, Bacterium gluconicum, Acetobacter ketogenum* and *Pichia Fermentans*. It contains vitamins B1, B2, B3, B6, and B12, as well as folic acid. Other good acids include glucuronic acid, which is important in the body to build polysaccharides such as hyaluronic acid vital for connective tissue; chondroitinsulfat acid which is the basic substance in cartilage; mukoitinsulfat acid which is good for our eyes; and also heparin and lactic acid for the colon.

These acids bind to toxins in the body and are then flushed out. Kombucha helps prevent the formation of certain cancers, helps with kidney and bladder function, helps to lower blood pressure, works well with weight loss, assists to regulate high glucose levels, and maintains proper blood sugar balance. It also softens veins, helps eliminate wrinkles and brown spots, reduces hot flashes, and is said to alleviate insomnia, chronic constipation, and help arthritis. There are many more benefits from this mushroom, not mentioned here. I have firsthand knowledge of this tea, as I have used it and made it at home myself. Look for a website about Kombucha Tea in the reference pages or go to *cajunernie.com* for a starter mushroom and recipe.

TEAGA TEA

A new product on the commercial market, but one that's been around for quite some time, is Teaga Tea. Teaga, also called Tiaga, is a bracket fungi containing germanium, found by Russian scientists to contain the highest amount of naturally occurring germanium of all the medicinally useful foods that support superstrong immune systems and better health. Until recently, this herb was not known for its great ability to support our immune system. The use of Teaga in America goes back to the

Northern Plateau Native Americans who observed great health when it was used. These Native Americans were bypassing such diseases as the plague, smallpox, and other life-threatening illnesses due to their strong immune systems. It was not until 1995 that these Native people were given tribal permission from their elders to release their long-held secret.

Teaga Tea does not cure anything by itself, but assists the body in healing itself. It does this by supporting increased liver function and the production of natural steroids which have antiaging, anti-inflammatory, anticancer, and antimutagen properties. It also increases oxygen catalysis (accelerates chemical reaction) resulting in a healthier body and increased energy. Teaga also has dietary fibers that are antiaging, which assist the body in removing toxic substances.

Teaga Tea has been said to stimulate the body to produce up to 4,000% more healthy neutrophils than the amount we normally have. These go into the bloodstream to fight infection. Neutrophils have been noted to bring about miraculous regeneration of damaged tissues and help to eliminate natural invaders in the body and, if abundant enough, attack cancer cells and other pathogens.

The following benefits of Teaga Tea have been observed by researchers:
1. Increased liver function
2. Anti-inflammatory properties
3. Normalization and regulation of insulin production
4. Stabilization of blood pressure
5. Antitumor and cancer benefits
6. Prevention of bacterial infections
7. Healthy immune system
8. Pain reduction
9. Assisting the body to remove toxins

The benefits of this tea are many, and testimonials from people who have used this herb show remarkable and incredible results. I have heard of amazing results from this bracket fungi, have used it myself and plan to use it again. This product is prepared by Life Research.

HEALTHY COFFEE

There are many coffee drinkers out there who really love their coffee but know they need to quit or reduce their intake. Try this new great tasting coffee to help you cut down, or stop. It is known as Gano coffee and is called the "healthy coffee." "Gano" is short for ganoderma (Ganoderma lucidum), a variety of mushroom. Ganoderma is known by different names around the world—linzhi in China, youngzhi in Korea, and reishi in Japan. Gano coffee has just recently reached the American market. It is a premium Brazilian coffee, which is blended with ganoderma and is not decaffeinated but is naturally very low in caffeine, low in acid, and has an excellent taste and aroma. Remember, most coffee is very acidic, high in caffeine, and is not good for the body, especially if you're watching your pH levels because of health problems.

Be very careful with the types of decaffeinated coffee you drink. Many of them contain formaldehyde, which is used to remove the caffeine, and is very toxic to your body. Formaldehyde is a carcinogen. Herbal teas and *Mat'e* tea are also very good substitutes for coffee.

Although there are some 200 species of mushrooms, ganoderma has the highest therapeutic value. For thousands of years, this herb has been highly regarded by the Chinese as the "miraculous king of herbs" and now has been added to premium quality Brazilian coffee beans.

Studies show certain types of mushrooms help the body strengthen itself, fight off illness, restore its overall balance and maintain natural resistance to disease. Reports show ganoderma has helped inhibit growth of malignant tumors, is an anti-inflammatory agent, antioxidant, antiviral, and helps lower blood pressure. Additionally, ganoderma strengthens the body's immune system, strengthens the organs for waste elimination and detoxification, increases brain power, provides more energy and vigor, decreases fatigue and rejuvenates you to make you feel more alert. It contains calcium, iron and phosphorus, as well as vitamins B, C, D, and pantothenic acid, which is essential to nerve function and to the adrenal gland.

All this and you can still have a great cup of coffee. If I drink coffee, which is very, seldom now, I use Gano. It has great taste without the jitters of caffeine. If you insist on drinking coffee, make sure you match each cup with equal amounts of water to cut the acidity. I use half a package which makes a good cup of coffee. Look in the reference pages under coffee for more information.

NOTES

NOTES

PART 10

HEALTHY OILS AND BAD OILS

THE GOOD AND THE BAD

In the mid 1950s, a brilliant German scientist by the name of Dr. Johanna Budwig discovered that by using a combination of flaxseed oil and sulphur-based proteins, and returning to the natural ways of eating, cancer could be cured. By "natural ways," Dr. Budwig meant recognizing the dangers of commercially manufactured dietary fats such as margarine, hard shortening, and vegetable oils. She preached against the use of fats and oils that have been hydrogenated or partially hydrogenated.

These oils are called "trans-fats," and are known as the artery-clogging oils. These oils are unnatural, and are produced by hydrogenating unsaturated fatty acids. This kind of oil has been around for the last 100 years in the food processing industry. A whopping 90% of these oils are hidden in processed foods, and are especially high in foods such as fried chicken, french fries, potato chips, cookies, cakes, and doughnuts, and not just the margarine that was supposed to be good to eat when I was growing up many years ago. We should be eating real butter, not margarine. Most margarine is100% hydrogenated oil and can do a lot of harm to our bodies. Do your best not use these types of oils at all.

Studies show trans-fats lead to a major increase in cancer, arthritis, diabetes, fatigue, heart problems and nearly all chronic illnesses. Absolutely avoid "Trans- Fats" also called, trans-fatty acids meaning, "partially hydrogenated oils." Children and adults who are overweight from eating these types of foods have displayed signs of insulin resistance, and this is what puts them at a much greater risk of developing diabetes.

Recent studies show over 16 million Americans have diabetes, which is becoming an epidemic, largely due to the shift in our food choices. Watch the movie *Super Size Me*. It's a real shocker. Trans-fat intake raises bad cholesterol (LDL) and also lowers good cholesterol (HDL). For this reason alone, trans-fats are accountable for tens of thousands of heart attacks each year. Substituting foods high in trans-fat for food containing pure polyunsaturated fat could reduce the risk of type II diabetes by some 40% as well as protecting against numerous other diseases. Soybeans are high in polyunsaturated fats (oils) which help lower the blood cholesterol level.

There are good fatty acids in our diets called "lipids" (essential fatty acids). These are the building blocks of fats and oils. There are also bad oils in our diet called "partially hydrogenated" (trans-fatty acids). Don't get these two mixed up.

How did these bad oils (fats) get into our food chain? In 1905, a well known American food company started making cottonseed oil. One of these products, Krispo, quickly caught on. The name was changed to Crisco and it soon became a household word. In 1907, this company, with the help of a German chemist, developed methods to make hydrogenation. They combined hydrogen atoms and fatty acids. This process made cottonseed oil into solid oil. This new modified (distorted) oil is now referred to as trans-fat, trans-fatty acids, hydrogenated and partially hydrogenated oils.

These oils change the protective barrier around the cells in our bodies, impairing them. This protective barrier is what protects our cells from damage. These trans-fatty acids are now hidden in thousands of our food products we eat every day. This causes our systems to be out of balance and we become sickly from a substance that is unknown to our bodies.

According to *www.fugitt.com/bb_0525.htm,* research shows trans-fats cause non-insulin-dependent type II diabetes and increase the risk of coronary heart disease, cancer, and auto-immune diseases. Over 100 studies show the harmful effects of this oil on our bodies. This kind of research has been suppressed for years and the public is more confused and misinformed as little bits of evidence begin to circulate. My question is why? Why does our government let this happen when the FDA and the Federal Trade Commission (FTC) are regulating our foods? I feel that modified foods like these should be outlawed for human consumption unless the manufacturers label them as trans-fats and state that these modified fats may kill you if consumed over time.

Our cells require true polyunsaturated, live electron-rich lipids, known as Omega-3 essential fatty acids (EFA), such as those found in raw flaxseed oil. The ancient Greeks and Romans used flaxseed oil in their diets. We have to obtain this oil from the food we eat. Alpha-linolenic acid (ALA), found in Omega-3 oil, is essential to many of our bodies functions if we want them to work correctly. It gives us smooth skin, increased healing abilities, and vitality. It also helps with reducing tumor growth, blood pressure, water retention, and a whole lot more. We also need two other types of Omega-3 acids we can only get from fish, which are eicosapentaenoic acid (EPA) and docosahexaenoic acid (DHA). These two Omega-3 acids are used directly by the body. ALA goes through a chemical change in the body to perform the same function as DHA and EPA if we are not getting enough DHA and EPA in our diets or with supplements. We have to be very careful when picking the correct fish to eat because many of our fish are now contaminated with toxins such as mercury, lead, and other deadly chemicals. Most Americans are deficient in these important fatty acids.

Today, flaxseed oil is regarded as high-quality oil. In Europe, people are using this oil for the prevention and treatment of all kinds of diseases such as cancers, tumors, arteriosclerosis and many others. Now, in the United States and around the world, people are discovering the benefits of flaxseed oil. The American Cancer Society says one in eight women will contact breast cancer and suggests that, "every woman take at least one tablespoon of 'lignan-rich flaxseed oil' daily to reduce her risk of breast cancer and minimize the potential for it to spread, should it occur."

THE BUDWIG DIET

Dr. Budwig, in her continuing research with oils and her search for a cure for cancer, went on to discover an all-natural way for people to replace important nutrients their bodies need in their daily diets by simply eating the "Budwig Diet." This diet is a combination of one cup organic low-fat cottage cheese and two to three tablespoons of flaxseed oil with highest lignans. These must be mixed before you eat them to be effective, since each triggers the release of certain properties of the other. I added this diet to my food intake diet and it helped to rid my body of cancer. For men, I have found out that freshly ground flaxseed is better. Recent studies have shown that flaxseed oil in men may cause problems with the prostate. Personally, I used this cancer diet every single day for two years while fighting cancer but my prostate had already been removed. Check out other foods that can be added to the Budwig Diet in the reference pages. A great flaxseed oil product that I use is called "Barlean's Fax Oil with Highest Lignan Content." When opening this bottle make sure to mix up the lignan that settles to the bottom. I use a table knife to reach the bottom of the container then shake it up to mix it in. If used daily, all you need to do is shake the bottle a few times to mix before using.

Dr. Budwig claimed this diet would prevent and cure cancer. She said, "The absence of linol acids (in the average Western diet) is responsible for the production of 'oxydase,' which induces cancer growth and other chronic disorders."

Take a quick look at breast cancer and compare Asian and American eating habits. Asians eat a diet consisting of foods such as rice, vegetables, and fish almost daily. These are all low in saturated fats. It is well documented that when Asian women eat an American diet, their rate of breast cancer goes up considerably. Studies show a link between the high-fat American diet and cancers of the colon, breast, gallbladder, pancreas, prostate, uterus, and ovaries. This *does not* mean we should cut "essential" fats out of our diet at all. And it *does not* mean that the less fat you eat the skinnier you will become. We need fat in the form of fatty acids free of toxins.

Essential fats are said to encompass the outer membrane of every cell we have. A deficiency in these good fats puts us in danger of disease. When we eat good fats such as olive oil, flaxseed oil, fish oils with EPA and DHA, such as cod liver oil, omega-3 and other fatty acids, even in small doses, our stomachs release a hormone that lets the brain know we are full. Without the good fats, our stomachs might be full of food, but we may still feel hungry and overeat. To be healthy and manage our weight correctly, our bodies need fats which supply us with essential fatty acids. This, in turn, will boost the fat-burning potential in our body and significantly reduce our bodies weight (fat) by using our stored fat for energy.

On the other hand, studies are now showing, even good oils are better for some people than others. The use of oils can be complicated when cancer is involved. Flaxseed oil is high in Alpha-linolenic (ALA), which studies are showing can be good in preventing breast cancer but is potentially a problem for men as a risk for prostate cancer. Raw flaxseed helps build a strong immune system. Flaxseeds, unlike the oil, are not as high in ALA. What I do to make sure I get omega-3, is buy the flaxseeds, grind them up in a coffee grinder, then sprinkle a large spoonful over whatever I'm eating. I also buy empty vegetarian capsules that I fill myself with the ground-up flaxseeds. I then take four of these capsules a day. This will allow me to get the ALA I need without taking too much of the oil itself. These empty capsules and flaxseeds can be purchased at your local health food store.

CONJUGATED LINOLEIC ACID (CLA)

CLA belongs to the essential fatty acid group of oils called Omega-6 acids which are rich in nutrients. CLA was first identified in 1987, at the University of Wisconsin-Madison, by Dr. Michael Pariza, Ph.D. Extensive research now shows this oil plays a very important role in our health. Studies worldwide are showing CLA helps protect against breast cancer, asthma, atherosclerosis, and clogged arteries, and provides allergy and blood sugar control (diabetes).

Linoleic acid, a natural part of pure safflower oil, is now processed into CLA. Research shows this oil helps our bodies use our existing fat to produce energy and increase lean muscle tissue. This process naturally shapes and slims down our bodies by taking off inches without drugs or chemicals. It helps the body metabolize existing fat deposits which are returned to the tissue through the bloodstream and used as energy. Studies also show it helps with type II diabetes by decreasing triglycerides, insulin, and leptin, and improves glucose utilization. Further studies are being done on CLA for the role it plays in fighting against cancer and atherosclerosis, which is a form of arteriosclerosis. An article in Woman's World December 16, 2003, magazine claimed that clogged arteries are also helped, and CLA may cut harmful LDL cholesterol by 10 points, and artery-clogging triglycerides by 50% in 12 weeks.

Omega-6 performs very important metabolic functions in the body. A two-year study in the April issue of the *Journal of Nutrition* said long-term supplementation of CLA is safe and well tolerated. It shows CLA decreases fat body mass and maintains lean body mass. This helps considerably with weight management by consistent reduction in weight and avoiding ups and downs of gaining and losing weight. Mark Cook, Ph.D., of the University of Wisconsin stated, "And now we know that CLA also helps replace that fat with muscle."

Research at the University of Wisconsin also shows CLA helps with asthma because it can slow or prevent lung inflammation triggering wheezing, difficulty with breathing, and respiratory distress. And when talking about breast cancer, Mark Cook Ph.D. said, "CLA blocks prostaglandin formations so cancer cells can be seen and destroyed before they've had time to grow." Oncologist Delbert Dorscheid, M.D., Ph.D., at the University of Chicago stated, "CLA can help prevent and even treat many of today's most frustrating health problems." CLA is available at your local health food store.

It is said the ratio of eating omega-6 to omega-3 should be 1 to 1 and no more than 3 to 1. People are eating way too much omega-6 oil, mainly in the form of unsaturated oils (bad oils) in ratios sometimes 50 to 1. We need to eat more fish or start taking fish oil supplements to help compensate for this problem. Cut way back on the amount of omega-6 oil you are consuming and start consuming more omega-3 from fish oils. If you're not careful, this *will* turn into a major health problem for you when eating too many unhealthy foods.

Alkylglycerlol (AKG) is another beneficial oil. This oil is found in shark liver and is a super immune system stimulator known to help fight cancer and other diseases. Shark liver oil has been used by the Europeans for a couple of centuries. It contains vitamins A, D, and E, omega-3 fatty acids, and other nutrients but is mostly known for the alkylglycerol and squalmine. Both are said to have medical healing properties. These two nutrients are said to help fight cancer of the lungs, breast, brain, and skin by stopping the tumors' blood supply.

COCONUT OIL

Coconut oil, which has been frowned upon since the 1960s, and had been labeled "bad oil," is now getting the recognition it deserves, and is said to even be superior to olive oil. What wasn't reported was the fact that the coconut oil used in these older studies was hydrogenated and not virgin coconut oil.

By now we should all know hydrogenated oil is not good for us. So why don't we all do an oil change for better health! The May 20, 2003 edition of *Women's World* called virgin coconut oil a "miracle food," and said it helps the body burn unwanted fat, triples your energy, lowers blood pressure, and greatly helps with thyroid problems. But always make sure of the purity of the oil you chose. To help lose weight with coconut oil, take one tablespoonful in the morning and another in midafternoon. Do this every day for a month to see the results. You should start to notice some weight loss within the first few days. Check to see if coconut oil is good for your blood type.

During the no-fat craze, saturated fats (oils) were labeled bad and were to be avoided. However, saturated coconut oil is of the medium fatty acid variety, digests easily and is used by the body in a different way than other oils. Other fats are stored by the body's cells, but coconut oil is sent directly to the liver where it is converted into energy, thus putting less strain on other organs. Coconut oil will speed up your metabolism and you will burn more calories. This will help you lose weight more quickly. Studies have shown unsaturated fats can cause hypothyroidism and lower your metabolic rate. Coconut oil is rich in lauric acid, which is an antibacterial and antifungal agent, and is used by the body to make monolaurin, the same monolaurin babies get from mother's milk to fight diseases.

There are three types of saturated fats in coconuts. They are short-, medium-, and long-chain-based oils depending on the number of carbon molecules they contain. Two-thirds of these three contain medium-chain. The medium-chain fatty acids are very healthy and may help your body lose weight. Coconut oil is processed by the liver and used as energy while stored in body fats. Coconut oil is said to speed up your metabolism so your body will burn more calories and have more energy.

Coconut oil helps to regulate blood sugar, and raises the metabolic rate, which stimulates an increased production of needed insulin, and increases glucose, which helps type-I and type-II diabetics.

These are only some of the great benefits of this oil. Make sure it's pure. Pure virgin coconut oil doesn't contain any of the dangerous trans-fats found in vegetable oils, margarine, shortening, and others oils. Coconuts are low in carbs, high in protein, and filled with nutrients such as calcium, magnesium, potassium, folic acid, and B vitamins.

NOTES

<u>NOTES</u>

PART 11

———•—

IMMUNE BOOSTERS

Immune boosters are nutritional products, vitamins, minerals and amino acids. The nutritional foods we eat are essential in our immune performance. Malnutrition can happen fairly quickly with all the bad food options we have to pick from these days. Usually, unless we are very health conscious, we don't stop to think about what we're eating before we eat it. Once in a while, we think about what we ate earlier and if it really was what we should have eaten.

It is true, the older we get the wiser we become. Living a happy life, with exercise, is a very important aspect of a healthy body, mind, and spirit. Below are a few important products for boosting the immune system and also foods and lifestyles that will weaken your immune system.

Boosting the immune system	Weakening the immune system
Greens	Overuse of sugars
Vitamins/Minerals	Excess alcohol consumption
Carotenoids	Food allergies
Bioflavenoids	Wrong type of fatty acids (fat)
Garlic	Lack of sleep
Selenium	Junk foods
Omega-3,-6,-9 fatty acids	Processed foods
Probiotics	Dead foods (no nutritional value)
Seaweed	Over-the-counter drugs
Herbs	Prescription drugs
Oxygen	Smoking

Also, teas and green food concentrates are excellent for the immune system and are talked about in this book. A few others that I have used for boosting my immune system are listed here.

DMSO

DMSO (Dimethyl Sulphoxide), is said to be a superb cancer-fighting product, and gets right into the cancer cells, killing them. It is especially effective when used with cesium chloride. In 1968, E.J. Tucker, M.D., and associate A. Carrizo, M.D., wrote an article regarding DMSO. They found that both DMSO and cesium chloride could target cancer cells and bind to toxic chemicals if used together. This product is mentioned in the Alternative Therapies in part 16 of this book.

DMSO is a nontoxic, 100% natural substance which comes from trees and is a by-product of paper. DMSO stimulates the immune system and scavenges hydroxcyl radicals, the most potent of the free radicals that cause damage to our bodies. It can also decrease the energy level of cancer cells and cause them to become benign. *Never* use DMSO without checking with a naturopathic or alternative physician.

IMMUTOL

A super immune booster you need to look at is "Immutol." This immune supplement is believed to be up to 200 times more active than the leading herbal immune system boosters. Hundreds of scientific studies have verified that the ingredients in this product have the ability to activate our immune systems safely and naturally. If you suffer from a weak immune system and are always sick, tired, or weak, you may want to try this product. A weak immune system may lead to, or you may already have, a problem like chronic fatigue, Epstein Barr, herpes, HIV, bacteria, fungis, cancer, or many other problems.

COLLOIDAL SILVER

Before antibiotics came along, one of the germ fighters doctors depended heavily on was silver, either silver colloid or silver salt. Silver colloid has the ability to kill bacteria, and is now used in some water purification systems and to help burn victims recover faster. Read the book, *Colloidal Silver, A literature Review,* by John Hill, D.C. Silver was used 1,200 years ago by Egyptians, Romans, Greeks, sailors, and then by the pioneers who populated our country. They used it for various illnesses and to keep their foods and liquids from spoiling. Prior to 1938, before antibiotics, colloidal silver was used by doctors as their main substance to fight bacteria in a more natural way than through the antibiotics they use today.

Antibiotics can harm our kidneys and liver functions. Colloidal silver promotes healing. These silver colloids are a mixture of very tiny particles of silver, as small as 0.01 microns in size, and suspended in a liquid form. Colloidal silver works against fungis and viruses, and accelerates healing. It is an allergenic, resistant to pathogenic strains and does not react with other medicines or herbs. It can also be used against cancer, as a preventative for many diseases, and as a booster of the immune system.

Dr. R. Becker, author of *Body Electric*, said that he believed a silver deficiency is the reason for the improper functioning of the immune system and silver is crucial for the destruction of bacteria and viruses. He went on to say silver regenerates tissue and eliminates cancerous cells as well as eliminating other abnormal cells. And, in the presence of silver particles, cancer cells change back to normal cells regardless of where they are in the body.

Dr. Bjorn Nordstrom, of Sweden's Karolinska Institute, recorded that he cured patients who had been designated by other doctors as "terminally ill" using colloidal silver. Read about colloidal silver, you will be impressed. One good website about this product is: *www.krchealth.com/colloidal_story.htm.*

OXYGEN SUPPLEMENTS

Oxygen supplements are becoming more and more important in our world. Clean oxygen is something our bodies need desperately as our planet becomes more and more polluted. The biggest user of oxygen in our bodies is the brain, along with the liver, which uses it to detoxify our blood. Other great benefits includes boosting our energy.

We get 90% of our energy from oxygen and 10% from our food and water intake. Two hundred years ago we were breathing up to 40% oxygen. Today it's much less, only about 20%. It is very important that we get more oxygen in our systems to help our bodies run smoothly. We also have the extra burden to deal with of bad diets and pollution in the atmosphere. Oxygen, as you know, is critical for all life to exist and an oxygen supplement is a very important part of good nutrition. Dr. Arthur C. Guyton, M.D., has said "All chronic pain, suffering, and diseases are caused from a lack of oxygen at the cellular level."

Dr. Spencer Way, M.D., said in the Journal of the American Association of Physicians, "Insufficient oxygen means insufficient energy that can result in anything from mild fatigue to life-threatening disease. The link between insufficient oxygen and disease has now been firmly established."

Believe it or not, oxygen supplements now come in a liquid form and in small bottles capable of being carried around in a pocket or purse.

One significant discovery of the 20th century is liquid "aerobic oxygen." This type of oxygen supplement increases oxygen concentration throughout the body, helps to kill harmful organisms like bacteria and viruses, all disease, boosts the immune system, and is a natural detoxifier for the body. It controls bacteria, not only in the body, but in your food and water, when added, and can be used along with brushing your teeth, as a mouth wash to kill bacteria in your mouth and gums.

Unlike drugs and antibiotics with there side effects, aerobic oxygen will not harm good bacteria, which is what we need to retain in our bodies for good health. When we are deficient in oxygen, our cells start to look for other forms of energy, like sugar, and our systems become acidic. This lack of oxygen causes our systems to produce improper chemicals, which weaken our cells and immune systems and lead to the deterioration of our bodies. Other severe health problems may follow, such as cancer and other diseases, if not corrected.

Aerobic oxygen is an alkaline product. It is not similar to, and should not be compared to, products such as oral hydrogen peroxide or chlorine dioxide which are acidic in nature. As you know by now, it is very important to keep your bodies alkaline. This is one of the great benefits of aerobic oxygen.

Have you ever really felt refreshed after a thunderstorm? The lightning from these storms charges up oxygen molecules in the rain, creating a negatively ionized atmosphere. Aerobic oxygen contains these negatively charged electrons, which attach themselves to the oxygen molecules. The ability to harness these negatively charged electrons in aerobic oxygen sets it apart from other products on the market. People who have worked up to 20 drops, three times a day, have reported great benefits from problems such as:

1. Lack of energy
2. Asthma
3. Emphysema
4. Chronic fatigue syndrome
5. Joint pain
6. Headaches
7. Poor circulation
8. Fibromyalgia
9. Sinus infections
10. Bronchial infections

Learn more about this product at: *www.natural-health-solutions.net* or go to your computers search engine or my website toward the back of this book. For more immune support you can also try: *www.immunesupport.com.*

<u>NOTES</u>

NOTES

PART 12

---·•·---

PARASITES, INTESTINES, AND A TOXIC ENVIRONMENT

PARASITES: WE ALL HAVE THEM

Another problem we have related to cancer is parasites. We all have them in our bodies, big or small, even if we don't have cancer. There *is* a way to kill these parasites and get on our way to healing ourselves. We're not accustomed to thinking about a total cure for cancer. I feel we are conditioned by the medical community to think only of a possible cure. Are the medical professionals and pharmaceutical companies trying to get us to think of remission as the only chance of ridding our bodies of cancer?

A great book to read, study, and order from is called *The Cure for All Cancers,* by Hulda R. Clark, Ph.D., N.D. She has done extensive studies on parasites that are causing cancer and disease in our tissues and organs. Dr. Clark has found evidence of parasites in every type of cancer to base her findings on, regardless of the type of cancer. In her book, she talks about parasites that can cause life-threatening problems when left untreated. These parasites can be passed between humans, by the food we eat, the pets we keep, the solvents and cleaners we use, and the lifestyle we choose to live.

A buildup of isopropyl alcohol in your body can invite unwanted guests (parasites) into your liver to make their home. When this happens, your immune system will lose the power to kill them and they will begin to multiply. Dr. Clark stated that isopropyl alcohol is found in 100% of cancer patients.

This alcohol is commonly used in cosmetics, shampoo, hair spray, mouthwash, body lotions, shaving supplies, rubbing alcohol and other products. Make sure to check the labels on all products for isopropyl alcohol. Clark also showed a way to rid your pets of the same parasites in this same book. When doing her studies, she set a goal of 100 patients to be cured of cancer before her findings were published. Her mark was met and passed in 1992, and she said, "The discovery of the cause and cure of all cancers has stood the test of time." In July 2004, I started on her herb recipe to rid myself of parasites. Go to the reference pages under Books, or go to: *www.you-are-what-you-eat.com/the-cure-for-all-diseases.html.* Also look into a product called Clarkia as a parasite cleanser. The ingredients include; *green* black walnut hulls, wormwood, and cloves. Clarkia is an herbal blend, in tincture form. I have used both the tincture form and capsule form. These can be ordered from her website or purchased at your health food store. Clarkia can also be found on the website reference pages in the back of this book.

IN TODAY'S WORLD

In today's world, anyone who wants to be healthy and live a well-nourished and longer life can do just that. You need superior nutritional products to start with. It's like getting a great tune-up for yourself, helps cell efficiency, and discourages disease.

Whether you're killing parasites, detoxifying your body of chemicals, or using herbs and whole food supplements, remember, they are not all equal. Purchase nutritional products of the best quality from the start so you get the proper nutrients your body needs. These supplements can be inexpensive insurance for you and have enormous health benefits. Choose wisely when picking out these products so you're not wasting money on something that's not going to work as well or something which only has a pretty label. Do your research or ask the employees in the nutrition stores for help in choosing the correct products. Don't try to guess at what products you need. You could be wasting your money. But one thing is for sure—now is the time to get serious about your health. Don't wait until something goes wrong. The time to start is now!

Remember, the cells of a healthy body are alkaline and the cells of a diseased body are acidic. Some diseases used to take a long time to show themselves, but now, as our daily diets are changing to acid-forming foods and drinks, disease is becoming a younger person's problem. Lifestyle is one major reason disease is now showing up earlier and earlier in all ages. This is a scary thought, but it's true. Your pH can be corrected and you can start to restore your health. Take the first step and check your body's pH level with a quick and easy test strip. You can find this at your health food store or drugstore, or you can find information in the reference pages of this book.

Today's Western medical philosophy preaches that if we have a disease due to some kind of outside germ, virus, or other influence that makes us sick, we can regain our health if we get rid of that germ or virus. So, using their logic, a bacterial infection should be fought with antibiotics and cancer should be cut out, poisoned, or irradiated.

If we must resort to antibiotics and other medicines, we need to put our bodies back in balance as soon as possible after finishing the medicine the doctor gave us. Otherwise, we keep weakening our bodies without rebuilding our immune systems. Additionally, when taking too many antibiotics, our bodies can build up a resistance and the medicine can become useless or less effective later when needed the most.

We are constantly being bombarded with mold, yeasts, microbes, and other environmental pollutants and toxins. Exhausts from cars and factories; smoke from cigarettes; household chemicals; preservatives and pesticides in our foods; chlorine, fluoride, and other toxins in our water; and other dangers that weaken our systems are some of these toxins. The key is to keep our internal environment balanced and nourished properly to start with, so those invaders can't take hold of us and start a disease.

HEALTHY INTESTINES

A healthy intestinal track will almost always contain 80% good and 20% bad bacteria. If we are taking antibiotics to kill the bad bacteria inside us, we are also killing the good essential bacteria that are keeping us healthy. We will need to help replenish the good bacteria by taking nutritional supplements such as acidophilus and probiotics. We can also eat cultured foods such as natural organic yogurts with no, or very low, natural sugar. These products contain active bacteria to replenish the good bacteria in our intestines. If we don't replace the good bacteria, more dangerous types of harmful bacteria can and will take over. Many times, the bad bacteria will be in the form of yeast.

Today, with our unhealthy lifestyles and bad eating habits, we are just the opposite. Our intestines contain about 80% bad, and 20% good bacteria. This can eventually lead to severe health problems such as candida (yeast overgrowth in both male and female), cancer, and numerous other diseases. In 1895, Louis Pasteur said on his deathbed, "I have been wrong. The germ is nothing. The terrain is everything." By *terrain* he meant the internal environment of our bodies.

Our small intestines can also build up mucus on the intestinal walls. Certain foods like pasteurized milk, milk products, and many cooked foods coat the villi. Villi are like tiny fingers that stick out from the intestinal wall to absorb nutrients from the digested food. The mucus builds up and sometimes becomes thick and blocks this absorption process. A colon cleanse can eliminate this problem.

A person with a severe mucus buildup could eat good foods and take great nutritional supplements, but could be starving his or her body because of very little or no absorption of nutrients. More pancreatic enzymes are now used to digest your food. When this happens, there are fewer enzymes left to help destroy cancer cells.

The cause of most nutritional disorders usually has something to do with our whole digestive system. Proper digestion, absorption, and assimilation are critical in our bodies for good health. Problems can arise from simply not chewing food long enough, to pH imbalance, not enough fiber in our diets, eating the wrong foods, or not taking proper nutritional supplements. If we can't digest our food properly our bodies will not get the proper nutrients required for regeneration. This will cause toxic chemicals to start forming. Eventually, our bodies will become weak. This can be corrected fairly easily if we catch the problem in time. If left untreated, it will eventually lead to serious problems, even colon cancer and other diseases.

If we have problems digesting foods, we need to change our eating habits. Most people eating the American diet don't produce enough hydrochloric acid for proper digestion. If we don't correct this problem, we are headed for major problems down the road. We need to cut out foods in our diet such as caffeine, and cut way, way back on carbohydrates, processed foods, sugars, and processed flour. These products can destroy B vitamins and deplete other important minerals we desperately need. Our stomachs use Vitamin B, minerals and enzymes to help make hydrochloric acid.

Think about switching to more raw foods. This means eat 80% raw vegetables, fruits and nuts, and 20% cooked foods. You can also steam your vegetables lightly to insure you don't overcook your food and kill the nutrients that are vital to your health. I understand many older people cannot digest raw foods easily. When I have digestive problems I take extra digestive enzymes during the day before meals. Vitalzyme is one good brand to use. Vitalzyme enzymes also help with inflammation and diseases such as arthritis.

If you have cancer or other diseases, or you are just trying to live a healthier life, you should definitely consider eating more raw food. If you have cancer, you should also consider not eating, or eating very few, fruits until your cancer is under control. Remember, fruits have fructose, which is a form of sugar. Cancer cells can also use this form of sugar to live on. Always think about what you're eating and start adjusting your diet to the 80/20 way of eating. This will keep you healthy and keep your body in an alkaline state. This is very important in order to live a healthy life and fight disease.

Our bodies make acid as a by-product of metabolism. We have very few ways of making ourselves alkaline unless we eat or drink the right types of food. All foods are either acidic or alkaline. Cooked foods are mostly acidic. Also, meats, eggs, breads, and sugars are acid.

Vegetables are mostly alkaline and fruits are mostly alkaline but some fruits such as lemons that are generally acidic have an alkaline effect on the body after being eaten except for blueberries, cranberries, and plums which remain acidic. It is important to remember I'm not talking about the acid in our stomachs. I'm referring to the pH in our bodies or our bodies' fluids, which is totally different. You can see a chart on this if you go to: *www.sagastevin.com/Articles/AnkalineDiet.html.*

Raw foods have all the vitamins, minerals, amino acids, life-essential enzymes and fiber that are extra important in keeping waste products from getting congested in the intestinal tract. If we do get congested, the food eventually turns toxic. These toxins back up into the liver and bloodstream, and continue being recycled by the body, causing other health problems. This can be one of the leading causes of cancer and other degenerative diseases. It is very easy to get confused with all our foods, wondering if they are acidic or alkaline in nature.

It is also hard to understand the need for acid in the body when I talk so much about keeping our bodies alkaline. Acid in the body is the key to great health. If we don't have enough acid in our stomachs, we accelerate disease. All foods that we eat and drink cause an acidic or alkaline body. The key is to eat enough alkaline foods to balance acidic foods. Eating too many acidic foods throws the body out of balance and our alkaline reserves will be used up to counteract this imbalance.

People with blood type O, like me, usually have more acid in their stomachs than the other three blood types and usually have an easier time digesting foods. When eating and drinking foods high in acid, such as coffee, our stomachs may have too much acid and we O blood types would probably be overacidic. Go to: *www.thewolfeclinic.com/acidalkfoods.html.*

If we eat the correct foods with the proper nutrients, our bodies will handle this without a problem. When we're not eating properly is when we start having problems. With low amounts of hydrochloric acid (HCL), foods are not digested properly and essential nutrients may not be absorbed.

As we get older, our HCL amounts start to decline. It is said that a low amount of potassium may result in low amounts of HCL and may lead to disease. As I have mentioned, cancer and other diseases have an extremely hard time living in an alkalinized environment. Almost all cancer patients have very high amounts of acid, called advanced acidosis. We do need HCL acid in our stomach to digest our foods. We also need to combat the acidic foods we eat with more alkaline foods to help keep disease away.

If you have a stomach ulcer or digestive problem and you're not digesting your food properly, you're more likely lacking HCL acid and pepsin. Instead of the food being digested by your body, the food rots, creating gas and organic acids to form. These acids start to eat away at the lining of your stomach. At this point, most people would reach for the antacids for relief, but this is only temporary relief. Taking antacids for this problem can actually make the problem worse. Antacids not only neutralize the acids of the rotting food in your stomach, but they also neutralize the digestive acids you need to digest the food. This can lead to serious stomach problems. You need to be taking digestive enzymes so your body can work properly.

It seems only natural to me that medical doctors would know how to explain this problem but, when I asked, they seemed to be unaware of the process or could not explain it properly, or maybe it was me. I finally had to ask a naturopathic doctor for help in understanding this complex problem.

ENZYMES

Digestive plant enzymes are essential in building and maintaining a healthy body. These enzymes help the digestive system break down what we eat, but are often destroyed by overcooking. Enzymes also help dissolve cancerous tissues. Today's scientists tell us dietary supplements containing the ten or more pancreatic enzymes are extremely helpful. These enzymes help us digest our food and can dissolve the protein coating of cancer cells, making the cells vulnerable to the attack of white blood cells. But remember, the majority of foods we eat today are overprocessed and result in almost total loss of enzymatic activity. This prevents digestion and the absorption of essential nutrients. As we get older, the digestive system becomes less efficient, which may lead to digestive problems and diseases such as colon cancer. As we grow, the body struggles for years to stay healthy despite the fact that we keep eating the wrong kind of foods.

Three types of these digestive enzymes, also called pancreatic enzymes, are extremely important to combat the intake of improper foods, as well as to digest all we eat. These three enzymes are *Proteolytic*, which digests protein; *Lipases*, which digests fat; and *Amylases*, which digests carbohydrates. Many of the enzymes in our foods die when cooked at or above 107 degrees, and almost all are destroyed at 140 degrees. Overcooking foods make them become very hard to digest, and can overwork the pancreas and digestive system, eventually causing problems. Toxemia is sometimes the result. Toxemia can lead to illness and disease in the colon. From the colon, it can move into the bloodstream, and eventually clog our arteries, and cause circulation problems and chronic fatigue.

Circulation is the only way the body's cells get the oxygen needed every second of the day. Without a sufficient supply of oxygen, our bodies become very acidic in nature. This can cause tissue degeneration, premature aging, disease, cancer, and over a long period, even premature death. Early signs of enzyme deficiency are gas, bloating, heartburn, stomach aches, feeling full when you're not, abdominal cramps, and unsatisfied hunger. These, and more, are some of the symptoms of enzyme deficiency, but they can usually be changed by taking enzymes and acidophilus, and by eating healthier. When all our enzymes are used up, working extra hard to digest the overcooked food, there are no enzymes left in the blood to destroy cancer cells. For optimum health, we must eat more raw, lightly cooked, or steamed vegetables. Enzymes are in most of our foods, but when processed or overcooked, enzymes die and we lose their benefits.

Normally, in a healthy body, 100 to 10,000 cancer cells are circulating inside us all the time, according to research done by Dr. Michael Williams. If our immune system is weak, cancer cells can attach themselves to an organ or tissue, and that's when we can be in serious trouble. Life cannot exist without enzymes. Those people who are deficient in these vital enzymes are very susceptible to physical problems, disease, degeneration, and early death.

A new generation of enzymes is called systemic enzyme supplementation. A product containing these enzymes is Vitalzym. It includes Serrapeptase, a type of Proteolytic enzyme which digests dead tissue, blood clots, cysts, and arterial plaque, and has all the benefits of other enzymes. Dr. Hans Nieper, a German physician, used seppapeptase to treat arterial blockage in his coronary patients. Studies show serrapeptase is also proving to be a superior alternative to the nonsteroidal anti-inflammatory agents traditionally used by doctors, such as aspirin, ibuprofen, salicylates, and naproxen. These are among the most common prescribed meds for inflammatory discomfort.

Many diseases, sometimes starting at childhood, could possibly have been avoided if parents had only known the importance of eating foods rich in natural enzymes. "Man is not what he swallows but what he digests and uses," Hippocrates.

PROBIOTICS

Probiotic is a word that means "for life." Probiotics are the beneficial bacteria in your intestines. They help support the healthy bacteria in your intestines and can improve your digestive system by helping it become more efficient. Probiotics also work by helping remove waste materials and toxins in your intestines and help the foods you eat digest more easily. If you're a meat eater who needs your protein, and are having trouble with digestion, try eating your green leafy salad after your meal, instead of before. This is because the carbohydrates in green leafy salads require less acid for digestion. By the time you finish eating your meat, the small amount of acid left in your stomach is sufficient to digest your salad.

Lactobacillus reuteri probiotics, (Lak-toe-bacillus-roy-tur-eye) occur naturally in your bodies and are the primary probiotics in your small intestinal track. It also can be found in mother's milk. It improves absorption of food, helps remove excess cholesterol from your blood, and stops the harmful growth of bacteria without interfering with the intestinal flora. *Bifidobacterium*, on the other hand, is the primary probiotic for the large intestine.

Keeping a balanced intestinal tract is very important in good health habits. When this balance is disturbed, so is your health. When probiotics get out of balance your immune system can be weakened. A poor diet plays a big part in an imbalance in bacteria.

Antibiotic use, environmental toxins, and preservatives in our food can also cause an imbalance of the good bacteria in the intestines. There are some 500 types of bacteria in our system. The two mentioned above are the most prevalent. Studies show, as we age, we have fewer good bacteria and more bad bacteria. This is another reason we should always watch our diets and eat as healthy as possible.

FUNGUS, YEAST, AND MOLD

There is fungus among us. Many people have a big problem with fungus (fungi), yeast and mold inside as well as outside their bodies. These fungi, molds, and yeasts are called mycotoxins, which are now well documented and studied. Fungi and their toxins are major naturally occurring carcinogens and are found in the foods we eat. They can cause serious problems over time with numerous diseases such as candida, cancer and life-altering conditions.

The fungi in our bodies are fed by carbohydrates we eat. Fast foods and other foods such as breads, potatoes, corn, alcohol, and sugar are high in carbohydrates. These types of foods can feed mycotoxins and over time, if not corrected, can lead to cellular damage. These types of foods are commonly contaminated with fungi.

Fungi are parasitic and require sugar and carbohydrates for fuel to be able to live and spread in our bodies. Drug therapy is known to lower our immunity and make our bodies more acidic, which opens the gate to other problems. This usually begins a cycle of doctor visits and more medications. Most medications are acid-forming, which sets the stage for additional fungi growth. We are all exposed to diseases but whether we contract one in our life depends greatly on a strong, healthy immune system.

The late Milton White, M.D., believed that cancer is a chronic infectious fungal disease. He found fungal spores in every sample of fungus he studied. Author Doug Kafman says fungi in foods may play a big role in cancer and he has seen people become free of documented leukemia when their diet was changed.

Mycotoxin fungi can be found in grains such as corn, wheat, barley, sorghum, and peanuts which are often contaminated with cancer-causing fungal poisons called mycotoxins. One of these, called aflatoxin, is said to be the most carcinogenic substance on earth.

Some 50 years ago, Dr. J. Walter Wilson, in his textbook on mycology (mycotoxins) said, "It has been established that histoplasmisis and such reticuloendothelioses as leukemia, Hodgkin's disease, lymphosarcoma, and sarcoidosis are found to be coexistent much more frequently than is statistically justified on the basis of coincidence." Go to: *www.mercola.com/2003/may24/cancer_contagious.htm*. This is a good site. The title of the article is "Is cancer contagious?" Also, read the book, *The Germ That Causes Cancer*, by Doug Kaufmann.

Check out Agrisept-L on your computer's search engine, or go to: *www.collagendiet.com; www.nutribiotic.com* and *www.pureessencelabs.com* for a product called Candex. These two products are taken internally and are great for yeast and fungal infections.

Candex contains no antifungals, so it cannot damage the liver as antifungal drugs do. The most difficult aspect of controlling yeast is the strict diet one must follow. Stay with protein foods such as chicken and fish and lots of vegetables. Avoid anything made of flour, processed foods, all sugars and products with sugar in them, especially if you currently have cancer or candida.

A.V. Costantini, M.D., former professor at the University of California San Francisco Medical School and former head of the World Health Organization, has data showing that mycotoxins in our food supply can and do cause many forms of cancer, including breast and prostate cancer. These fungi come from the air and live in the mouth, sinuses, gut, vaginal tract, and other body cavities. This is an example of how necessary it is for our immune system to be in top shape all the time to protect us.

NOTES

<u>NOTES</u>

PART 13

ALTERING OUR FOODS

THE PROBLEMS WITH OUR (WHITE MUSTACHE) MILK

There are also chemical toxins in our milk. That's right! You should probably sit down while you read this. Our wholesome milk isn't all that wholesome. From what I've learned, milk is good only for calves. But in today's world it's not even good for them. With all the man-made toxins fed to and injected into cows these days, we should be running the other way. In 1992, the Consumers Union in New York found 52 different antibiotics in the milk we drink. Not only that, the milk we buy in our stores contains toxic chemicals that can do the body extreme harm. Most cow's milk, if not organic, contains pesticides, dioxins, herbicides, hormones, and antibiotics. This is just the start of it all.

Pasteurized milk is heated and held at 161 degrees F for a short time to destroy any harmful bacteria. Pasteurization, in addition to killing harmful bacteria, kills beneficial bacteria, enzymes, and phosphates needed by the body to absorb calcium. It also kills important minerals we need, which may contribute to many types of disease. Believe it or not, even in pasteurized milk, blood, pus, bacteria and viruses have sometimes been found in the past. Some of the best milk on the market, if you wish to drink milk, is organic and has been ultra-pasteurized.

Insulin-Like Growth Factor One (IGF-1) is a natural growth hormone found in both humans and cows. However, with modern dairy technology, many farmers have been injecting large numbers of cows with Recombined Bovine Growth Hormone (rBGH), approved for use in 1994 by the FDA. This is a genetically engineered bovine growth hormone. Injecting cows with rBGH increases milk flow by 10 times but is also said to raise IGf-1 in our bodies to dangerous levels.

Research is showing IGF-1 is a key factor in the rapid growth of prostate, colon. and breast cancers. It is now suspected IGF-1 is also responsible for other cancers. The rBGH chemical toxin is injected into about 10 million lactating dairy cows in America each year. The white mustache isn't that good for us after all.

When it comes to cheese, the Tillamook cheese company does not use cheese products with rBGH in it. Check out: *www.foxbghsuit.com/bgh4.htm* and *rense.com/general126/milk.htm.* These are two good sites that talk about milk and toxins.

Julian Whitaker, M.D. said, "Recent studies have found a seven-fold increase in the risk of breast cancer in women with the highest IGF-1 levels, and a four-fold increase in prostate cancer in men with the highest levels." Dr. Samuel Epstein of the University of Illinois, in his article in the International Journal of Health Science, clearly warned of the dangers of high levels of IGF-1 contained in milk from cows injected with (rBGH).

The growth Hormone rBGH is also in infant formula. If you are giving your child formula to drink, or if you drink milk yourself and are breastfeeding, your child may also be getting the rBGH hormone from you. Be careful, and think before you drink milk. Go to: *www.notmilk.com/drlarsen.html* and *www.notmilk.com/deb/100498.html* to find out more about this. These aren't the only two sites on milk and toxins. There are plenty to be found on the Internet or in the reference pages of this book.

Another word we know in milk processing is *homogenization.* Homogenization is a process that breaks down butter fat globules in the milk so they don't rise to the top. This process is done for convenience and to give milk a longer shelf life. Milk fat molecules contain a substance called xanthine oxidase (XO). This can be a problem if it is homogenized and has been linked to heart disease. These large XO milk molecules are broken down by the homogenization process into very small molecules.

Dr. Kurt A. Oster, chief of cardiology, Emeritus at the City Park Hospital in Bridgeport, Connecticut found that when milk is homogenized, some of the XO substance can pass through the wall of the intestine and into the bloodstream. The enzyme XO is found naturally in our bodies and helps the liver function properly. But if any XO from an animal like a cow enters into our bloodstream, it creates havoc within our arterial walls and can directly attack parts of the heart muscles. Plaque then starts to build up, and the thickening and hardening of the arteries starts, resulting in arteriosclerosis and the restriction of blood flow to and from the heart. This can result in heart disease, cancers, allergies, asthma, and desensitization to antibiotics. In 1983, Dr. Oster and Dr. Ross wrote *The XO Factor* and went into detail about this serious problem with homogenized milk. Go to *www.steroidology.com* and find out more about this. You can also find information through the search engine on your computer. Type in, "The Journal Atherosclerosis" (1989; 77: 251-6).

Just about the time you think there's no hope in drinking healthy milk, another product comes along. A great alternative for people who want to drink milk is whey. Whey is what forms at the top of the milk when it is not homogenized. A product called Whey Healthier, an organic milk product, is a drink mix high in protein that kids and adults love, and is said to be "whey" healthier than what we're used to drinking in the regular milk varieties. This organic product has no artificial sweeteners and is said to be free from all chemicals and hormones. Other whey products can be found in your health food store but, unless organic, may have other toxins already in the product that are not listed on the label.

Go to: *www.Mercola.com* and type in "Whey Healthier," or turn to the reference pages in this book. I am extremely careful when eating or drinking any dairy products and have cut dairy products almost completely out of my diet, except for the Budwig Diet talked about earlier. Every once in a while I'll eat some organic yogurt but to me, milk is a scary subject. Make sure you know what you're drinking and what you're giving to your kids to drink. It can make a huge difference in your health and your family's health.

Take a look at this scenario with the information you just read about milk. Add to that the problem with eating saturated oils (using the wrong type of oils, margarine, etc.), and eating the wrong foods (sugars, trans-fatty acids, processed foods, etc.). This mixture can cause serious problems to your health. Once in the body, these types of foods may not only put your body into a very acidic condition and may cause your blood to thicken but over time may start clogging up your arteries with cholesterol and plaque, which will raise your blood pressure and increase the workload on your heart. This buildup of cholesterol and sticky plaque on your arterial walls reduces the oxygen in your system and starts to create a condition called hypoxia. Remember, cancer thrives in an anaerobic environment—the less oxygen it has to deal with, the faster it can grow and spread. If you have cancer, or another serious disease, any reduction of oxygen in your system is detrimental to your health.

A cholesterol and plaque buildup may cause any of three types of arteriosclerosis, leading to balloon angioplasty and/or stents having to be inserted to hold your blood vessels open, a possible heart attack, or multiple bypass surgery down the road. Just one of these problems is bad enough for your body but, with two or more of these major health problems, you have an extremely dangerous situation. I think of it as a time bomb.

According to *Taber's Cyclopedic Medical Dictionary*, atherosclerosis, one of the three forms of arteriosclerosis generally recognized, is "the most common form of arteriosclerosis" and "the single most important cause of disease and death in Western societies." If you consider yourself in normal health, you may not have any of these conditions, but the majority of Americans have some degree of cholesterol and/or plaque, buildup in their systems and don't know it. Is this the road you're heading down, maybe unknowingly? It's time to get off that road as fast as you can.

LECITHIN CAN HELP

Cleaning the plaque out of your circulatory system is essential, whether you have cancer or not. A very easy and safe way I have found to melt the sticky plaque buildup out of my circulatory system is called the 12-day flush. I learned of this flush in a book written by Dick Quinn called *Left for Dead*. After having a heart attack and a failed bypass, he saved his own life and beat heart disease the natural way without drugs, as I did with prostate cancer.

Lecithin is a natural fat that breaks down fat and cholesterol, enabling the body to use what it needs and discard the rest. Lecithin cleanses the circulatory system, provides essential nutrients for proper function of the brain and nervous system, helps metabolize fat-soluble vitamins A, E, D, and K, prevents and breaks up gallstones, cleanses and improves liver function, lowers bad cholesterol (LDL), alleviates arteriosclerosis and clears up skin problems. Lecithin used to be extracted from egg yolks, but soybeans were discovered to offer a purer, more nutritious, and less expensive source of lecithin than egg yolks. Lecithin is a fatty substance manufactured naturally in our bodies and widely found in many animal- and plant-based foods, including eggs, nuts, whole wheat, wheat germ, liver, beef hearts, and soybeans.

Lecithin is produced daily in your liver, if your diet is adequate. It is needed by every cell in the body and is a key building block of cell membranes. Without it they would harden. Almost two-thirds of the fat in the liver contains lecithin. Lecithin protects cells from oxidation, largely composes the protective sheaths surrounding the brain, and makes up 30% of the dry weight of the brain.

Lecithin not only prevents cholesterol from building up on the arterial walls, but also helps remove deposits that have already formed. Normally, cholesterol dissolves only at a very high temperature, but when lecithin is introduced, cholesterol will liquify at a temperature lower than normal body heat.

Once dissolved, the scouring action of normal blood flow can wash cholesterol off the arterial walls. Held in suspension by lecithin, the newly liquified cholesterol can pass harmlessly through the body.

Scientists found that simply adding soybeans, the best available source of lecithin, to the diet reversed arterial heart disease, lowered genetically high cholesterol counts, counteracted the effects of a high-fat diet, and regulated blood sugar.

Lecithin is a major source of choline and inositol, B vitamins responsible for helping metabolize fat. Inositol stimulates hair growth and aids in digestion. Inositol and lecithin may benefit diabetics by helping to correct impaired glucose tolerance and keep insulin levels under control.

Liathinose, an enzyme produced by the body, unlocks the choline in lecithin. Choline is the catalyst that helps maintain a healthy liver. Choline is one of the few substances able to break through the brain blood barrier to stimulate the production of acetylcholine, a neurotransmitter. Acetylcholine is essential for proper brain function, enhances the operation of the brain, and stimulates the brain cells to produce more acetylcholine. Lecithin helps correct problems resulting from deficiencies of choline and other nutritional substances in the kidneys.

Although dietary lecithin is the primary source of choline, this nutrient is also available through food; it appears in high concentrations in liver, egg yolks, peanuts, cauliflower, soybeans, grape juice, and cabbage.

Some research indicates choline from lecithin may be able to boost memory, counteract depression, dementia and Alzheimer's disease, all traced to a deficiency of acetylcholine. Tardive dyskinesia, a disabling brain disorder caused by failure of the brain cells to release acetylcholine and causing involuntary body movements, is now routinely treated with choline and Lecithin.

Incidentally, choline taken alone has side effects not encountered with lecithin. Bacteria in some individuals break down choline. As a result, the choline is rendered ineffective and you will smell like a dead fish. I'll stick with getting mine from lecithin.

Multiple sclerosis has been linked to lecithin deficiency or depletion. The severity and frequency of attacks decreased when patient's diets contained lecithin or oils that stimulate lecithin production. Demographic studies have revealed areas with high-fat diets have a higher incidence of multiple sclerosis than areas where diets high in polyunsaturated fat were favored. Lecithin contains a high amount of linoleic acid, an essential fatty acid found in certain types of polyunsaturated fat. Linoleic acid in lecithin is theorized to account for the successful treatment of multiple sclerosis. Researchers have stated the essential fatty acids, such as linoleic acid, found in lecithin, are 50 times more active than those contained in other dietary sources.

Healthy skin thrives on proper use of fatty acids. Lecithin has been used successfully to treat eczema, seborrhea, psoriasis and certain types of acne. Since, because lecithin is a fat fighter, it targets bad fat in "love handles," "spare tires," and "cottage cheese thighs." As a natural diuretic, lecithin also eases water weight gain.

The ability of lecithin to emulsify fat also helps the body absorb fat-soluble vitamins A and E to help maintain a healthy heart. Vitamin E strengthens and rebuilds capillaries, keeps damaged tissue soft and flexible, inhibits the formation of blood clots, and increases the ability of the circulatory system to provide blood and oxygen to the heart while decreasing the heart's need for oxygen. Vitamin A helps reduce blood cholesterol levels and stimulates natural lecithin production.

There are many types of lecithin on the market. Which one is best? The quality of the lecithin supplement depends on the proportion of phospholipids it contains. Look for supplements with a phospholipid content of no less than 98% and a high proportion of phosphatidyl choline. Phosphatidyl choline approximates the kind of lecithin present in the heart. The higher the phosphatidyl choline content, the purer the lecithin supplement is.

Caution must be taken when searching for a high quality lecithin supplement. Label information on this supplement is more misleading than most any other. Beware of imitation granules that contain only about 30% lecithin.

There are a few tip-offs when trying to spot low-quality lecithin. For example, pure lecithin contains no protein. A label listing a calcium content of around 6% of the recommended daily allowance signals the presence of an additive like tricalcium phosphate. Additionally, pure lecithin doesn't absorb moisture rapidly so if the label reads "instantly dispersible" it may contain whey or milk solids. Pure granular lecithin, devoid of additives and preservatives, is the most potent source of lecithin.

Now for the "12-day flush," designed to clear our clogged arteries. Nutritionists recommend starting a lecithin regimen by taking three tablespoons of lecithin granules once a day for 12 days with light exercise about two hours after you take it. That's it! After cleansing the circulatory system, nutritionists recommend taking a tablespoon or two a day to maintain good health. Taking one tablet of garlic and one tablet of ginger each day with the lecithin will further assist softening plaque, clots, and cholesterol; however, you may not want to add these two if you are taking blood thinners.

Granular lecithin can be sprinkled on cereal, mixed in juices or hot drinks or eaten by the spoonful. My wife and I take our lecithin mixed with fruit juice. We add other herbs and flaxseed oil into the juice as well. We buy a bottle of organic juice that is low in sugar to mix our lecithin in. Remember, all juices have fructose, and cancer loves sugar. One juice I use frequently is called Just Black Cherry, by R. K. Knudsen. I drink 4 to 6 ounces a day for this mixture. This juice is very low in natural sugar. Add water if needed.

GENETICALLY ALTERED (ENGINEERED) FOODS

Genetically altered foods also called genetically engineered foods (GEF) have shown up in our stores and marketplaces without being noticed by the average consumer. Most of us don't have a clue about what these foods are, what or where they came from or when all this happened without our knowledge. But we do use them nearly every day. People have farmed for over 10,000 years without these food modifications.

In 1998, an independent research study was conducted at Rowlett Research Institute in Aberdeen, Scotland on genetically engineered foods and their effects. The tests showed evidence of organ, intestinal, and brain damage to animals that were used in this test.

GEF contain genes derived from bacteria and viruses. These changes in our foods are radical from traditional methods, yet sales of these new types of food are permitted without adequately informing the public, resulting in possible serious damage to our health. GEF contain genetically modified organisms (GMOs), animals and plants whose genetics have been altered to something which is not normal.

GEF is a process of artificially changing the blueprint of an organism and scientifically transferring genes from one organism to another. It is already known that we do have the ability to do gene transferring, which is another way to feed the world. However, some feel it reveals the commercial and political motivation for money and greed without regard to possible dangers to our population. Now, large chemical companies would like GEF seeds to replace conventional seeds. Just think, you could be growing GEF foods in your own garden at home fairly soon if this happens, and not even know it.

GEF's are becoming mainstream in foods such as breads, pasta, candy, margarine, meats, dairy, vegetables, and more. In a few years, it may be impossible to find natural foods unless you grow them yourself. One would think that the powers that be, in all of this, would be working on finding a way to fix our problem with our depleted soils and grow real organic food instead of GEF foods. Take action now so we can at least know what foods have, and have not, been altered by placing labels on products we purchase and feed our families with. If our food industry is going to make GEF, we need to have the right to choose what we're eating. Go to: *www.thecampaign.org.*

Our food industry and the FDA assume these foods are not substantially different from our existing foods. I feel this kind of altering of foods could never happen in nature so why mess with altering our foods and taking very big chances with possible side effects? Only a small amount of testing has been done on GEF so far. Who knows the impact these foods will have on us down the road? Remember to try and buy organic vegetables from local farmers if you can. Or you may be the guinea pigs.

Today, roughly 65% or more of all foods sold at your grocery store for your consumption have been genetically altered, without our knowing the effects these products will have on us before we consume them.

So far, it has not been required for the food industry to label such GEF foods. New laws need to be established requiring products that *have* been modified or altered in any way to have labels placed on the package before the product can be sold. It would only be fair for us as consumers to know what we're eating. Some foods in the health food section of your store, are starting to show up with labels on the package that show if the food you're about to purchase has been genetically altered; however, I have only seen very few of these kinds of labels. Check out; *www.gefoodalert.org* for a great cartoon explanation of this new type of food that you are already eating. Also, go to *www.inmotionmagazine.com/geff4.html* for the hazards of GEF.

MICROWAVING OUR FOODS

Microwaves are a form of electromagnetic energy. Microwaves are also used to relay cell phones, long distant telephone calls, television programs and computer information. Microwave energy is very fast, can travel at the speed of light, and can also cook our food. Unfortunately it cooks our food in a very different and much unhealthier way than conventional cooking does.

At present 80% or more of American homes have microwaves. It is said that the manufacturer of these types of ovens are suppressing the facts and evidence about the dangers of what microwaving does to our food. Because of this suppression of evidence, people keep using microwaves without knowing the dangers and complications microwaved foods are causing in our bodies.

Cooking our food using a microwave oven changes the molecular structure of the food by the radiation process. Radiation causes ionization. This happens when a neutral atom gains or loses electrons. In 1976, the Russian government banned microwaving. Do they know something we don't, or are we not being told the real truth about the dangers of microwaving?

In 1991, a hip replacement patient in the United States was given blood that had been warmed in a microwave for a blood transfusion and died when receiving the blood. Blood used for transfusions is routinely warmed but microwave ovens are not used to do this.

In the book, Health Effects of Microwave Radiation-Microwave, Dr. Lita Lee stated that, "every microwave oven leaks electro-magnetic radiation, which harms food and converts it into dangerous, toxic, and carcinogenic products." She went on to say, "Microwave ovens are far more harmful than previously imagined."

Further, she says microwaving baby formula converts certain trans-fatty acids into their synthetic cis-isomers. Studies show that synthetic isomers, whether cis-amino or trans-fatty acids, are not biologically active. Furthermore, one of the amino acids, L-proline, is converted to its D-isomer, which is known to be neurotoxic (poisonous to the nervous system) and nephrotoxic (poisonous to the kidneys). In her book, she says it's bad enough that many babies are not nursed, but now they are given fake milk (baby formula) made even more toxic via microwaving. It is recommended not to heat a baby's bottle in a microwave. The bottle may seem cool on the outside but the liquid may be extremely hot on the inside, burning the mouth and throat of the baby drinking it. Microwaving can also cause changes in the milk such as a loss of vitamins and minerals. Microwaving breast milk may cause it to lose its natural protective properties.

In *The Body Electric*, Robert O. Becker said, "Because the body is electrochemical in nature, the force that disrupts or changes human electrochemical advents will affect the physiology of the body." This is also discussed in, *Warning, The Electricity around You May Be Hazardous to Your Health,* by Ellen Sugarman.

German and Russian researchers who also investigated this say, *microwaves can cause cancer* and a large decrease in the nutritional value of food. This can cause destruction and disruption of biological processes and can destroy valuable cancer-fighting compounds also found in our vegetables. Microwaves break down human life energy and the energy field in our bodies. They also cause degeneration and circuit breakdown in the front portion of the brain, loss of balance, and the long-term loss of vital energy. Our bodies cannot break down the unknown by-products that are made while microwaving foods.

The Russian research on microwaving was published by the Atlantis Raising Educational Center in Portland, Oregon. It was shown that carcinogens were formed in virtually all foods tested. No foods tested were microwaved longer than necessary to be cooked properly. It was shown that:

1. meats were caused to form d-nitrosodientholamine, a well-known carcinogen;
2. milk and cereal grain amino acids were turned into carcinogens;
3. thawing fruits turned glucoside and galactoside into carcinogenic substances;
4. plants, especially root vegetables, were turned into carcinogenic free radicals;

5. essential vitamins and minerals were altered into compounds the body could not break down, which then rotted and turned into cancerous free radicals, causing stomach and intestinal tumors.

This may explain the high increases in colon cancer. Microwaved foods may cause a loss of memory, dizziness, headaches, stomach pain, and cancer, emotional instability, and numerous other complications. Microwaving also causes food molecules to change form into radiolytic compounds.

In 1980, Swiss biologist and food scientist Dr. Haus Hertel studied the effects of microwaved foods. He found that microwaving can cause a decrease in blood hemoglobin levels, white and red blood cell problems, altering of protein molecules and of LDL and HDL cholesterol levels, and possible altering of the structure of water when heated or boiled. Cells of nutrients can become destructively polarized, and free radicals can be created. This may cause major disruption in the human biological processes. This, in turn, may cause cancer-causing agents to increase and start to attack our bodies, causing disease. Many people, even after reading this, will continue to use their microwave because of the fast pace of the world we live in today and the convenience of it all. I hope this won't be you!

NOTES

<u>NOTES</u>

PART 14

TOXINS, DETOXIFIERS
AND CLEANSERS

SMOKING

Smoking is not only a very bad habit to start, it is one of the worst choices you can make for life. You are setting yourself up for a whole host of diseases and a life of very poor health and high medical bills. Smoking is extremely habit-forming and is the leading cause of many types of diseases. You're not only hurting yourself but friends and loved ones around you. Cancer kills hundreds of thousands of people each year, and a large number of these deaths are from smoking and secondhand smoke.

If you are fighting disease of any kind, with medication or nutrition, and you smoke, you're only fooling yourself. Smoking keeps your immune system run down so it can't do its job properly. One of the most widely used chemicals in cigarettes everyone knows about is nicotine. Nicotine is a poisonous chemical and is toxic. It is also used as an insecticide, so just who are the cigarette manufacturers trying to kill?

Smoking is also inflammatory to your arteries' interior lining, the endothelium. Each cigarette you smoke adds new damage and your blood vessels never have time to heal. This can start a fatty plaque buildup on your arteries' walls, not to mention the development of cancer. Smoking constricts your blood vessels and capillaries. This significantly reduces circulation in all your extremities. This, and a lack of exercise, are major contributors to hand and foot amputations in the elderly.

Smoking is like an injection of toxic chemicals into your body, and it drives these poisons directly into your brain and lung tissues. Smoking releases hundreds of toxic gases into your system, which do extensive damage such as depriving the body of vitally needed oxygen. Smoking also robs the bones of needed nutrients and can lead to male infertility, reduced mental function, birth defects, and cancer, to name but a few problems you may encounter down the road.

Each year more than 440,000 people die in the United States from tobacco use and nearly one out of every five deaths is related to smoking. Cigarette smoking accounts for 30% of all cancer deaths in this country and is the cause of cancers of the throat, lung, larynx, and esophagus, and contributes to some types of leukemia, and also to cancer of the colon, rectum, kidney, stomach, cervix, liver, uterus, and more. About 87% of lung cancer deaths are caused by smoking, and lung cancer is the leading cause of cancer among men and women. If this isn't bad enough, smoking is the major cause of strokes, heart disease, and bronchitis. It is also associated with sudden infant death syndrome (SIDS), stillbirth, miscarriage, and premature deliveries.

There are at least 4,000 chemical compounds in cigarette smoke and roughly 43 have been identified as cancer-causing toxic chemicals. *Hello!* If you want to live a good life, and give your body every chance to stay healthy, smoking is definitely not the way to go. Remarkably, the body can heal itself of the damages of smoking. Studies show that if you were to quit smoking right now, the inflammation in your body will start to recede, the risk of cardiovascular disease will decrease, and 15 years after you stop smoking your body, including your lungs, will be completely healed, aside from possibly permanent damage. Sometimes even damage considered permanent has disappeared. That is, if you haven't already contracted a serious disease or ailment from this killer.

If you continue to smoke while making positive changes in your other health habits, you seriously have very little chance of changing your body to be healthier even when taking nutritional products. Let me say it again. Smoking will inhibit any chance for your body to completely heal itself by keeping vitally needed oxygen from areas that need to be healed. This may advance to the point of serious disease, when you could have made a very big difference and remained healthy by not smoking. The chemicals, smoke and tar, you are inhaling can be your death sentence if you continue to smoke. I could go on and on but let's get on with the rest of this book. *Please* stop now while you still have a fighting chance.

CHEMICAL TOXINS IN OUR FOOD

Are the meat we eat and the milk we drink safe? Well, that depends on whether we listen to the U.S. Department of Agriculture (USDA), or a doctor of nutrition. In 1989, our country produced its one millionth man-made chemical. You may want to sit down as you read this part.

There are 70,000 or more man-made chemicals registered with the Environmental Protection Agency (EPA) and 65,000 of them are hazardous to your health. Volume 1, Number 1, of the *Prevention* newsletter 2005, said that, "6,000 new chemicals are being tested in the United States every week" and went on to say, "More than four billion pounds of toxic chemicals are released into the environment each year. Out of this 72 million pounds are known carcinogens." I would say, this puts us in somewhat of a fix. Think about what this is doing to the air you and your kids are breathing. These agents are listed under the broad term of "pesticides," which covers a very large group of toxic chemicals. When we are exposed to pesticides, our systems' natural functions can be interrupted and cause us to contact a disease. These chemicals build up in our bodies and are stored in our fat.

In 2005, a report from the Center for Disease Control's environmental health laboratory shows there are some 148 chemicals found in the blood and/or urine of people living in the United States. A similar test was done by the Environmental Working Group's Mount Sinai School of Medicine in New York. They found 167 industrial chemicals in nine volunteers. Out of these findings, 76 of the chemicals are known to cause cancer in humans; 94 are toxic to the brain and nervous system; 82 affect breathing and lungs; 79 are known to cause birth defects and 86 have an effect on hormones. They also found these toxins to be high in toxic metals such as lead, aluminum, and mercury.

Out of the 70,000 chemical combinations, some are called pesticides, insecticides, herbicides, fungicides, and parasiticides. We now use about 10 pounds of pesticides per year for every person in our country. These chemicals are used to spray on, and put in, the foods we eat and the foods we feed the animals (cows, chickens, pigs and others) that eventually wind up in our bodies for breakfast, lunch, or dinner. This does not take into consideration toxic chemicals from paints, metals, and acid rain. Our bodies are in a "toxic overload mode." It's no wonder that we're sick and dying. Think about it!

Dairy, meat, seafood, and processed foods all contain some form of industrial chemicals. Chemical additives, hormones, growth stimulants, antibiotics and other drugs are added for our "enjoyment." Wow, doesn't that sound appetizing? And to top it off, many of these chemicals have carcinogenic, neurotoxic, and immunotoxic effects on our bodies.

Let's take one great American food, the hot dog. This famous little piece of meat, if we should call it that, has nitrates added to it as a preservative. Nitrites are also added to lunchmeats and cured meats. When nitrates are added and this processed meat is cooked, carcinogenic N-nitroso compounds can be formed. Some of these can accumulate in our bodies, can cause cancer, and are risk factors for childhood leukemia and brain tumors. Most hot dogs also contain benzene, dacthal, dieldrin, lindane, hormones, and many other potentially harmful ingredients such as antibiotics which *do not* have to be listed on the package. "They" are not telling us "the whole truth, and nothing but the truth," about what's in these meats because there is no law that says "they" have to provide this information. Chemical additives are allowed by our food and drug laws to be combined and listed on labels as, believe it or not, "natural flavors," and so forth.

Recent research at Washington State University shows that exposure to environmental toxins does affect our health more than we knew. New research not only shows that our parents, and their parents before them were exposed to fewer toxins than we are today, but those same toxins from many past generations may all be passed on to us through our parents' genes. "These toxins may even modify our DNA. Low doses of toxic chemicals have a much larger impact on us than once thought," says Dr. Michael Skinner, one of the researchers on this important project. So, what should we expect for our kids?

There are also excitotoxins! These are aspartame (artificial sweeteners), as mentioned earlier, and monosodium glutamate (MSG). These are toxins that are put in our foods and drinks to enhance flavor. These two known chemical toxins, out of thousands, are a couple of the worst and yet the most widely used.

Research has shown many studies that link the use of aspartame and MSG to many common problems such as ADD, ADHD, dyslexia, depression, brain tumors, paranoia, reveal a special connection between multiple sclerosis and aspartame. Check out *www.mercola.com* and type in a search for *excitotoxins*.

Growing numbers of doctors and clinics are convinced that excitotoxins are causing numerous serious disorders. The amount of these toxins being added to our food since 1948 is astronomical. MSG alone has doubled every year and over 800 million pounds of aspartame have been consumed in various products since it was approved by the FDA. These two products are used in almost all processed foods, in our spices, yeast, soups, gravies, diet sodas and more.

These toxins react with brain receptors that destroy certain neurons by actually "exciting" them to death. During a lifetime of free radical injury, due to things like chronic radical injury, chronic stress, infections, and poor nutritional intake, the nervous system is weakened and made more susceptible to excitotoxic injury. This can lead to neurodegenerative diseases and can happen long before clinical diseases develop. It is well known that the immature brain is four times more sensitive to the toxic effects of excitatory amino acids than the developed brain. Again, we should be extremely careful with what we feed our bodies.

Many people, for some reason, don't think this applies to them. They think, and even say, "I haven't done anything wrong to have all these toxins in my body." Well, it's not that you have done anything wrong—it happens to you by just living your daily life in the polluted world. Your world has changed drastically from when your parents grew up and will change that much more in the future. Look around and see what's going on around you. Step outside your comfort zone and get involved. Now is the time to start. Everything you eat, everything you drink, everything you put on, or rub into your skin, needs to be looked at again. It's the fingernail remover and the hair spray you are using. It's the aluminum in your favorite tooth paste and antiperspirant. Stop, think, and change your life. Read the ingredients on all products you buy *before* you purchase them and ask yourself if you really need or want to put that in or on your body.

OUR BLOOD AND TOXINS

We are bombarded with toxins every way we turn. We come into contact with thousands of chemicals and toxic metals every day. They are in the air we breathe, the water we drink, the foods we eat, our over-the-counter medicines and the prescription medicine we take (pharmaceuticals). We also get toxins from the vaccinations we receive from childhood, into adulthood. Surprised? Well, it's true. Even the flu shots people think to be safe contain mercury, formaldehyde, and a few other toxins.

Studies show we have at least 400 to 800 toxins in our fat, tissues, and organs which can put our bodies into a toxic overload. These toxins can do damage to different areas of the body. One place where toxins do serious damage is the receptor sites used for absorbing our essential minerals in the intestines. When this happens, over time, it may cause all types of serious health problems.

A toxin overload can eventually damage the brain, cause auto-immune problems, cancers of all types, nutritional deficiencies, heart disease, Lou Gehrig's Disease (ALS), which my father had, MS, Parkinson's, schizophrenia, and the list goes on.

Roughly 20 million pounds of mercury are estimated to flow into our oceans each year. This is only one toxin and it is one of the worst. It causes the fish we eat to have mercury in their meat which is passed on to us, the consumers. Penguins in Antarctica and polar bears in the arctic are now being found to have mercury toxins in their bodies. This is one of many toxins spreading throughout our oceans today. In

1974, the World Health Organization said that 60% to 80% of environmental toxins contribute to many of our diseases. This is one very big reason why we need to detoxify (cleanse) our bodies.

Herbs such as black dogwood, golden flower and white elk, and supplements such as lecithin, are some of the excellent blood purifiers and can do wonders for our systems by cleansing the liver. Toxins can be found in every part of the body. Once the colon is overloaded, and we don't get rid of these waste products, the colon can dump toxins into the bloodstream. Once in the blood, the toxins travel throughout the body, build up over time, and cause many other health problems. It is extremely important that we eat the correct types of food and always drink plenty of fresh water. If we don't, we will eventually pay the price, one way or another. I'm sorry to have to be the one to inform you of these terrible problems but try and remember, *I did have cancer.* That's why I wrote this book, to remind myself, and to let you know, of the dangers for you and your families.

OUR LIVER

The liver is the super-heavy-duty cleansing unit for our bodies. It continuously cleans our blood, creates bile to carry toxins out of the blood, and helps to neutralize toxins it removes from our blood. The liver is also the major fat-burning organ in the body. Every minute of the day our blood passes through the liver to be cleansed and sent back into the bloodstream. The liver also maintains and balances our hormones, helps with proper digestion, controls our cholesterol, and stores vital vitamins and minerals for our bodies to use on demand, to mention just a few of the functions it performs.

When the liver is not running properly because of too many toxins or an insufficient nonnutritional diet, we may start to experience that "run-down feeling." Our muscles and joints may become tender, stiff, and hurt and swell from these toxins we eat, breathe, drink, and sometimes soak into our bodies from cleaners, chlorine, fluoride, drugs and so forth. When this happens, an overgrowth of yeast can attack the liver and slow our systems down. This can make the immune system run sluggishly and leave it wide open for other viruses and germs to settle in.

Michael T. Murray, N.D., author and respected authority in natural medicine, talks about herbs that have a beneficial effect on our liver function. One of these, and one that is very impressive in this process, is an extract of the herb called milk thistle, also known as silymarin. Silymarin is of the flavonoid family and protects the liver from damage and also helps with the detoxification process in the body. Silymarin acts as an antioxidant, which helps protect the liver from toxic chemicals. Silymarin has shown to be effective in treating liver disease. It is said to also help with the inflammation and the solubility of the bile duct which, in turn, has a positive effect on eliminating gallstones from the liver. Find out more in *"Ask the Doctor, Nature's Liver Remedy: Milk Thistle Extract."* Look this up in the reference pages under pamphlets.

We need to help our whole bodies stay healthy so they will last us a lifetime. There are many liver-cleansing products on the market today that can cleanse the liver and make our lives and bodies much healthier. Milk thistle, lecithin, dandelion root extract, artichoke extract, and turmeric extract are a few of the herbs and supplements that play a major role in cleansing the whole body. By cleansing the liver, we also cleanse our blood.

Elson M. Haas, M.D., founder and medical director of the Preventive Medical Center of Marin and author of several popular health books said, "Through my 25 years in medical practice and health care...I have come to believe that the cleansing and detoxification process is the missing link in Western nutrition and one of the keys to real healing. I have seen hundreds of patients over the years transform regular or persistent illness into health and greatly improved vitality."

Find a good parasite cleanse, a kidney cleanse, a liver cleanse, a gallbladder flush, a colon and bowel cleanse, circulatory system cleanse (mentioned later), and a general body cleanse. Parasites can live almost anywhere in the body and thrive in our colons and organs and grow bigger from acid-forming foods such as sugar, processed and junk foods. As they grow bigger, the toxic waste they expel will make us sicker and more toxic. A kidney cleanse is done mainly to cleanse the tubes and tissues of toxins which have collected in the area. The colon cleanse is said to help reabsorption of water and nutrients that we desperately need and to eliminate the film that has built up on the intestinal lining.

This film covers the villi, used by the body to absorb nutrients from the food we eat. All of these help to remove toxins and restore health. Remember that fiber plays a crucial part in a healthy colon.

Colon problems can start with deficiencies in plant fiber. We can increase the amount of fiber in our diets by eating properly with more vegetables and fruits. This can drastically reduce the onset of problems such as diverticulitis. When doing a colon cleanse, make sure fiber is added.

Check out *www.bodypurenow.com* for detoxifying body pads. These pads are great to use on your feet and should be applied at bedtime. They can be placed on other areas of the body as well, during the day or at bedtime. When applied to the feet, the pads work with our meridians (energy flow) and organs in our bodies like the principles of reflexology. These pads draw out toxins through the pores of our bodies. Extensive work in Japan by research scientists, backs up the claims for these toxin-eliminating pads. This is a simple and effective way to remove toxins from our bodies. I use them myself.

Look for these at your health food store or go to the website mentioned. If you really want to be healthy, detoxing and cleansing the body is a must. Get your body revved up and running correctly. Keep it that way by changing your eating habits for life. Watch your energy skyrocket and the extra pounds fade away. Remember, I am not a doctor. This is part of what I have learned to stay healthy. Always check with your doctor or medical practitioner first. Also, read about zeolites for detoxifying, coming up next.

NATURAL CELLULAR DEFENSE (ZEOLITES)

As Paul Harvey always says, "Stand by for the News"! To keep it short, let me say, "Zeolites are amazing minerals." I learned about this product in January, 2006. There is a U.S. patent on this product, number 6,288,045 which was approved in September 2001, two years after my surgery. This natural product was submitted to the U.S. Patent Office under the title "Epithelial Cell Cancer Drug." The word "drug" is given to any product approved by the FDA whether it is a natural product or not. The name of this product is "Natural Cellular Defense"

(NCD), which is formulated using zeolite technology and sold by a company called Waiora. Unfortunately, this product was not on the market when I found out I had cancer. I wish it had been.

NCD, also called Cellular Zeolite is a 100% natural liquid supplement. Dr. Harvey Kaufman has spent some 37 years of research to formulate this natural product. His original plans were to continue with the drug approval process but found it to be very time consuming and eventually introduced his product to Waiora's scientific advisory board. They soon found this product could be available to the market much sooner as a natural supplement and at a much lower price.

Zeolites were first discovered in 1756 by Axel Fredrick Cronstedt, a Swedish mineralogist. He discovered a form of this mineral called stilbite and noticed it lost water when heated. He gave this mineral the name zeolite, which is Greek for boiling water.

This NCD formula is a negatively charged volcanic mineral formula that works at the cellular level removing toxins and heavy metals from our bodies. The negative charge of the zeolite molecule will not reverse polarity or dissipate while in use. It would have to be heated to 900 degrees for days to break apart or melt.

Zeolites are negatively charged particles of glass-rich volcanic rock and sea water and are able to travel through the body with their negative charge and remove heavy metals that have a positive charge. These particles do this by binding and trapping them together in its structure of honeycomb-shaped particles, flushing them out of the body.

A recent study was done by the Environmental Working Group which is a non-governmental organization that provides the public with new, locally relevant information on environmental issues. In this study the Red Cross collected blood from 10 umbilical cords of newborn children to check for toxic chemicals. The results from this test showed there were 287 industrial chemicals, toxins, and pollutants found in the blood of each cord. From this test, 180 of the toxins found were cancer-causing toxins, 217 were toxic to the nervous system and brain and 208 were toxins that cause birth defects in animals. Also, toxic heavy metals such as mercury, lead, and aluminum were present, along with pesticides and herbicides which are also very toxic. If this doesn't scare you, I don't know what will.

This form of zeolite has been labeled 100% safe by the FDA. NCD is now sold as a natural supplement and not as a drug. The Waiora Company, which sells this supplement, makes no claims that NCD will cure anybody of any disease.

In an interview Dr. David Graham, the individual who blew the whistle on Vioxx and its harmful effects, and was responsible for its removal from our stores' shelves, said that NCD showed 78% full remission for stage 4 cancer, in one of the company's studies. This study was on 65 people, with various types of cancer, with a prognosis of two months to live. One year later 51 people, in this study, were still alive and cancer free, a 78% cure rate for this group. The study was conducted by the researchers at LifeLink Pharmaceuticals in the state of Ohio and was one small study by this company.

This product has shown to act as a tumor suppresser and may stop the growth of tumors by directly suppressing growth signals, acts as an antioxidant, fighting free radicals that may cause damage to DNA. It also traps and kills nitrosamines (a toxin found in lunchmeat, hot dogs, etc.) in the intestines, removes heavy metals from the body, acts as an antiviral agent against infectious disease and other threats to the body such as the bird flu. It also improves the absorption of nutrition and helps to balance pH levels in our bodies, to mention a few great benefits.

Zeolite also activates our body's P21 gene, which kills cancer. It acts as a tumor suppressor and appears to stop the growth of tumors. The trimetallic part of the zeolite molecule crosses the nucleus of the cancer and destroys it. Research shows this form of zeolite works on receptor sites and cell wall membrane proteins. It does not affect ordinary, healthy cells at all.

The next few paragraphs are what I have read on this product from the U.S. Patent Office. The patent number assigned to this product on September 11, 2001 is 6,288,045 and can be found at this government website: *www.uspto.gov.*

After reading the U.S. Patent on this epithelial cell cancer drug, I found that research shows:

- Zeolites kill cancer cells and do not affect or kill healthy cells.
- The zeolite's composition is synthesized from naturally occurring nontoxic zeolites. Studies used in the Patent say, "The composition is synthesized from a naturally occurring nontoxic zeolites and has a 100% kill rate within 72 hours against buccal mucosa and ling squamous epithelial cell cancers. It is not cytoxic to healthy human cells." Epithelial cells are skin tissues that cover and line the body. They cover all our organs and cavities, such as inside the chest and abdominal cavities. Epithelial cell cancers are called carcinomas and make up 85% of all cancers. The compounds of the present invention are particularly useful in treating these epithelial cell cancers in mammals.
- The present compounds may be particularly useful for the treatment of solid tumors for which relatively few treatments are available. Such tumors include epidermoid and myeloid tumors, acute or chronic. Such tumors also include nonsmall cell, squamous, liver, cervical, renal, adrenal, stomach, esophageal, oral, and mucosal tumors, as well as lung, ovarian, breast, and colon carcinomas, and melanomas (including amelanotic subtypes). The present compounds can also be used against endometrial tumors, bladder cancer, pancreatic cancer, lymphoma, Hodgkin's disease, prostate cancer, sarcomas and testicular cancer as well as against tumors of the central nervous system, such as brain tumors, neuroblastomas and hematopoietic cell cancers such as B-cell leukemia/lymphomas, myelomas, T-cells leukemia/lymphomas, small cell leukemia/lymphomas, as well as null cell, sezary, monocytic, myelomonocytic and hairy cell leukemia.

NOTES

<u>NOTES</u>

PART 15

OTHER PRODUCTS, METHODS, AND PAIN KILLERS

GREAT PRODUCTS AND ALTERNATIVE METHODS

Here are some other great cancer fighters that are definitely worth looking into. These are natural products I have not used, but are products for fighting disease and improving your health. So, for me, the search goes on. I feel very fortunate to have found all the products in this book, many of which I continue to use today. All the products listed below are said to be great cancer and disease fighters.

1. AHCC. This product contains several species of medical mushrooms.
2. Anvirzel. An herbal extract good for cancer and AIDS.
3. Arginine. An amino acid essential for life. Inhibits the growth of tumors.
4. Artemisinin. A Chinese herb, called sweet wormwood.
5. Betaine. A by-product of sugar beets which may help kill cancer cells.
6. Cancell. A liquid electrolyte formula. Safe, and is said to be very effective.

7. Carctol. A combination of herbs from India, treating all types of cancer.
8. CoQ10. A vitamin-like natural substance used for many diseases. Great for cancer.
9. Epican Forte. Vitamin C, lysine, proline, and high-potency green tea with 80% polyphenols.
10. Far Infrared Therapy. A method using "far infrared heat" to kill cancer cells.
11. IP6. A nutritional supplement with B complex and inositol.
12. MGN3. A natural immune enhancer.
13. Methyloglyoxal. Selectively targets cancer cells without hurting healthy cells.
14. MSM. An organic sulfur compound made from DMSO.
15. Mycosoft Gold. Immune enhancer from medical mushrooms.
16. N-Tence. South American healing herbs.
17. Oxy E. Cellular oxygen enhancer.
18. Poly-MVA. A powerful nutritional supplement.
19. Soil-based organisms. Find information on your search engine at: *critters, soil-based organisms and immune function.*
20. Tian Xian. A combination of 15 herbs.
21. Proxenol. A product containing high amounts of *Morinda citrifolia*, also found in Noni juice.
22. Digestinol. A product containing high amounts of aloe mucilaginous polysaccharides. A concentrated product of the aloe vera plant.
23. E-Tea. Essiac Tea herbs in capsule form.

You can also find more information about nine strategies to help kill your cancer at *www.cancer-prevention.net*. This is an excellent website. Take the time to read and understand all the information on it. Pour yourself some herbal tea, sit back, take a deep breath and settle in to read this great cancer information. This is not a site to skim over.

Don't run off after reading that site. Another great article to read is *www.mercola.com/article/sugar/sugar.htm*. It's only one or two pages long.

NATURAL PAIN KILLERS

There are many great natural pain killers on the market today. They not only kill the pain but also help with the inflammation in your joints. Some of the better natural pain-killing supplements I have found, and use when needed, are:

1. Arthritin. A good product for arthritis and joint pain.
2. Flexitol. A natural ingredient that addresses the whole body.
3. DLPA. Research indicates that DLPA can fight chronic pain, mood swings, and premenstrual syndrome; increase energy and mental alertness; and help with attention deficit hyperactivity disorders.
4. Arth-X. This product helps with bone, joint, and ligament pain. It also has minerals and trace minerals which help with swelling of joints.
5. Freederm AC. This is a rub-on lotion, with emu oil, that is known to ease muscle and joint pain, including arthritis. It also contains oleic acid, which has an anti-inflammatory effect on the body.
6. Biofreeze with ILEX. This is another rub-on lotion that works great against back, neck, joint, and muscle pain.
7. Easol. This is said to be the only natural health supplement pain reliever that includes a complete list of botanicals in one supplement. Easol may relieve chronic pain from numerous conditions.
8. In-Sync. This is an alkaline-forming formula of 39 natural ingredients that are all tried and true. This is a very good pain killer.
9. Formula 303. This is a maximum strength natural relaxant for muscle spasms, tension and stress. It works great.
10. ArthroZyme. This is a proteolytic enzyme and is effective with joint and cartilage functions. I experienced that this product helped me with inflammation and pain.

There are many natural and alternative pain killers, these are only a few. You can also ask an alternative doctor or go to your local health food store that carries these type of products.

<u>NOTES</u>

NOTES

PART 16

---·◆·---

ALTERNATIVE THERAPIES
AND PRODUCTS

CHIROPRACTIC

Chiropractic health care is one alternative therapy I would not be without. It has saved me from an operation and has relieved and eliminated severe and crippling pain in my lower back and sciatic nerves in my legs. I am deeply grateful for chiropractic therapy.

The first recorded chiropractic adjustment was made in September, 1895 by Dr. Daniel David Palmer. He opened his first chiropractic school in 1897. By 1902, 15 students had graduated from his school, now called the Palmer School of Chiropractic. Doctors of chiropractic are trained to analyze your spinal column. It is said, from the chiropractic perspective, a poorly functioning spinal column is the cause of many different ailments which, left untreated, may lead to disease.

From my experience with chiropractic therapy, when pain is present there are great benefits this alternative health care therapy can give in addressing your overall health. Your spinal column has billions of nerve fibers. These fibers send energy and messages to every part of the body. If you are misaligned, and have blockage of nerve function along your spine, this can lead to nerve damage, which can lower resistance to the organ connected to a particular nerve. This can cause sickness and disease.

Chiropractic care is a wonderful option in staying healthy and pain free as I have done for years. Doctors of chiropractic will work with you so you may become pain free, without prescription medication. Believe me, this really works.

THERAPEUTIC MASSAGE

This type of therapy is found in all civilizations, from the ancient Greeks to the Roman baths and on to today's massage therapists. The hands-on therapy of massage relieves stress and tense muscles, reduces anxiety, relieves blocked energy flows throughout the body and also complements numerous other health care therapies such as physical therapy and psychotherapy. It works excellently in conjunction with chiropractic care.

There are several types of massage, from a light invigorating massage to a deep muscle massage that works out sore and injured muscles. I always take the time to see a massage therapist first before a chiropractic treatment. I believe these two therapies work extremely well together. Find a doctor of chiropractic and a massage therapist you can talk to and feel comfortable with. You will be amazed what they can do for you. I find it much better to use these two therapies together rather than using prescription or over-the-counter drugs.

ACUPUNCTURE

Acupuncture is a method of Oriental medicine that is totally different from the Western style of medicine. The traditional Asian or Eastern style of acupuncture is based on the ancient Chinese theory of the flow of qi which nourishes the body through distinct channels. Acupuncture adjusts this flow of energy where it is insufficient and drains it from other areas where it is not needed, thereby restoring balance to the body, helping with pain and swelling, and promoting and reestablishing the free flow of qi. Acupuncture can also cure problems in major body systems such as respiratory, gastrointestinal, circulatory, urogenital, gynecological, musculoskeletal, psycho-emotional, and neurological disorders.

The first time I saw how acupuncture actually worked, I was very pleased with the results. When my son was two years old, he was having difficulty breathing through his nose and had to breathe only through his mouth most of the time, especially at night when sleeping. My wife and I took him to an acupuncturist because all other prescription medicines had failed to help and our medical doctor seemed to be at a dead end except for prescribing more medication and/or surgery. After his first visit, he slept throughout the whole night, breathing only through his nose, with no difficulty. This made me a true believer in what acupuncture could do.

MEDICAL OZONE THERAPY

This type of therapy has been used as a cancer treatment in Europe for a hundred years or so, and is now here in the United States. It is said there are over 3,000 medical references in Germany showing the effectiveness and safety of ozone treatment. There have been over 50 years of recorded treatments on humans with extraordinary results and millions of dosages given to patients. It's all about oxygen concentrations in our blood. Ozone is extremely safe, very effective, with no side effects.

The German Medical Society on Ozone Therapy says, "Ozone has proven to be the safest medical therapy ever devised." Considering about 100,000 Americans a year die from drug reactions and interactions, ozone therapy is amazingly safe. Ozone therapy must be used with other therapies, since not 100% of the cancer cells are killed. Now, we don't have to travel far to have this treatment done. We have clinics right here in our country. You need to read this website. It's impressive. Look in the reference pages under Medical Ozone Therapy.

CHELATION THERAPY

Chelation therapy is another great natural way to detoxify and clean the blood. As I noted earlier, we all have large amounts of toxic metals and chemicals in our bodies which may eventually cause cancer and other problems. Chelation therapy is administered into the body by intravenous drips and can take several treatments to help cleanse the blood. A blend of magnesium, B complex, amino acid, and other natural acids such as ethylene, diamine, tetra, and acetic are sometimes used, along with other vitamins and minerals. Chemicals and heavy metals enter the body over a life span of normal breathing, eating, drinking, cooking, going to the doctor and dentist, and the bad habits we pick up over the years such as smoking, drinking, drugs, and so forth. Chelation is a great way to relieve our bodies of possible current and future problems. Chelation also improves metabolic function and blood flow by cleaning blocked arteries.

CESIUM CHLORIDE

Nature's most alkaline mineral is Cesium. In 1984, Keith Brewer, Ph.D., treated 30 patients with various types of cancer with cesium and the results worked: All 30 patients survived their cancer. Cesium starves cancer cells by diminishing their fermentation, and raises a person's alkaline (pH) level to the range of 8.0 or above. This neutralizes the lactic acid in the body and stops pain within 12 to 24 hours. People living in parts of the world with a high cesium content in the soil do not contract cancer.

When toxins weaken our bodies, the immune system is greatly compromised. Our body loses the ability to exchange oxygen and our cells go into survival mode. This starts a fermentation process of the cells, starting formation of cancer cells. Once the fermentation starts, it is nonreversible, even for new cells that are forming. The cancer cells grow out of control and must be destroyed, the sooner the better.

With immediate help you can start to turn this problem around. Since cesium has a high pH value when taken internally, the life of the cancer cells is short. Within a matter of days, the cells start to be killed and the body fluids start flushing out and eliminating the dead cancer cells from the body. Read the book, *Cancer Cover-Up*. Do not take cesium without first talking with an alternative doctor.

UKRAIN

Naturopathic, alternative, and other doctors and practitioners overseas are saying a product called Ukrain is the single best anticancer agent used to date. They say that unlike chemotherapy, Ukrain kills cancer cells but does not hurt normal cells. Ukrain was developed in 1978 by Dr. Wassyl J. Nowicky, director of the Ukrain Anti-Cancer Institute of Vienna, Austria. He brought out his findings in August 1983 at the 13th International Congress of Chemotherapy.

This compound is derived from a plant called "greater celandine" *(Chelidonium Majus L.)*. This plant has a unique poppy like look that selectively kills only cancer cells and does no harm to the body's defenses, but actually fortifies the immune system. It can even be beneficial when used with cancer medications, if those are even needed at all. It is toxic against cancer, at its therapeutic dose, and encapsulates larger tumors through anti-angiogenesis. This cancer therapy is said to be expensive, about $10,000 to $20,000 a year, with intravenous injections proven to be the best method to be used at this time.

This herb contains alkaloids such as chelidonine, which are said to kill cancer cells. Other plants, as well, are known to have alkaloids, but Ukrain has herb and druglike compounds that work together and seem to have a strong affinity in killing cancer. As many as 149 scientists from 16 countries and 47 universities have done research on Ukrain and have published their findings on this cancer therapy.

Ukrain is patented in both the United States and Europe and has many scientific studies to prove its efficacy. Check out *www.ukrain-drug.net/webspreed/s001.htm* for a lot more information on this product. This site says "Ukrain could replace chemotherapy in treating almost all cancers," and "Cancer can be reversed." Check for websites and phone number on this product in the reference pages.

CYTOLUMINESCENT THERAPY (CLT)

CLT is a fairly new therapy on the horizon and one that is showing great results. It is said to be one of the most promising therapies for the near future and the next generation of Photodynamic Therapy. A CLT light-sensitive drug (agent) would be injected into the body and attach itself to the tumor cells or be injected directly into the tumor. When exposed to this light the CLT begins to produce oxygen. Tumors normally grow in an environment void of oxygen. The oxygen kills the tumor.

The CLT Institute, based in Killaloe, Ireland, the original CLT location, is already using CLT on patients with great success. Dr. Porter, who runs this clinic, is mainly responsible for the endoscopic light process that is used.

Fotoflora, a photosynthesizing agent, is one of the two drugs used in this therapy and is a plant-based photosynthesizer. The fotoflora light process can reach a depth in the body of 9 centimeters, or 3.5 inches, and when used on both sides of the body, can reach almost everywhere needed. Photofrin, an animal, blood-based product is also used. Photofrin can reach a depth of 1 centimeter, and is mainly effective for small skin cancers and certain other internal cancers reached with this endoscopic light.

It is said that all types of cancers can be eradicated by using CLT, with little or no problems of scarring. There are also indications that it is useful in treating AIDS, cardiopulmonary diseases, eye diseases, and other diseases as well. CLT seems to be a very promising aspect in the fight against cancer and other diseases. Look for cytoluminescent therepy or CLT on your computer's search engine for more information that may have come out recently.

Q-RAY IONIZED BRACELETS

These are stylish wrist bands for men or women which work great for pain. People who wear these ionized bracelets say, "The moment you put one on your wrist you will start to notice a difference in your level of pain. Research at the Mayo Clinic is showing results to be no different between wearing placebo and ionized bracelets.

It is said positive and negative ions ease pain of the energy flow in our bodies. Most people when asked if the ionized bracelet really works or not say they would not take it off because of the relief they got when wearing one. My wife, who has shoulder pain, gets results when using this product. If you have pain, try it out.

MAGNETIC THERAPY

While western Europe and Russia have been using magnetic therapy for some 30 years, it seems our researchers have not had many clinically sound studies on the great benefits of magnetic therapy. There is growing evidence that the magnetic field of magnets has a beneficial influence on the physiological processes of our bodies. There is a wide array of magnets on the market today. Results are showing magnetic therapy can be quit dramatic for pain relief for some people and subtle for others.

<u>NOTES</u>

<u>NOTES</u>

PART 17

HEALTH HABITS, PRODUCTS, AND DIET

WHAT I DO FOR GREAT HEALTH HABITS

Here are 23 things I did for great health while fighting my cancer, the same ones I follow today.

1. I use a pH test strip to see where my acid/alkaline level is. This is a very simple test strip that shows me if my body is alkaline or overacidic.
2. I started a whole-food liquid vitamin, mineral, and oxygen supplement lifestyle.
3. I started juicing every day or stopping at an organic juice bar whenever possible.
4. I stopped drinking soda pop, diet pop, diet or sugar waters, and juices with added sugars.
5. I keep bottled water around to grab instead of pop or sweetened juice.
6. I drink only organic milk if I drink any at all, and I eat free-range (organic) meats, poultry, eggs, and vegetables. This is very important.
7. I started stretching and exercising for better health and to help chase away stress.
8. I made nutritional products, whole food supplements, and organic foods a priority in my life.
9. I stopped eating sugars and junk foods, (processed cookies, cakes, donuts, chips, etc).
10. I stopped eating fried foods, processed foods, and fast foods.

11. I stopped holding on to anger and grudges I had. I let them go and now feel a difference in my health.
12. I do something good for myself and my family every day.
13. I tell someone I care about, every day, that I love them, and mean it.
14. I am now much more of a happy and positive-thinking person. This alone has a big impact on your health.
15. I stopped eating and cooking with the wrong types of oils. My family and I use pure olive, coconut, flax and macadamia nut oils. These are excellent oils to use and cook with. Remember, essential fatty acid oils are good and trans-fatty acid oils are bad.
16. I stopped using alcohol and tobacco products.
17. I breathe deeply and fill my lungs completely, with fresh air several times a day. Let the oxygen in. First, blow out the old stale air all the way, and breathe in deeply filling your lungs completely. Oxygen is extremely important for us to be healthy. Then find a good liquid oxygen supplement to use like the one I mention in this book.
18. I started a body, cleansing routine with Essiac tea and plenty of water.
19. I consulted a homeopathic doctor who specializes in this field.
20. I stopped using artificial sweeteners of all kinds, in drinks, gum, breath mints, candy, and food.
21. I got off all sugars, processed foods and grains, which are high in carbs.
22. I think about everything I put in my mouth before I eat, and what I'm going to be eating later. Have a plan.
23. I stopped using all aerosol can sprays, regular lotions, rubbing alcohols, toothpastes, and regular store-bought sun screens, and switched to all natural products. I also stopped using household cleaners, switching to natural cleaners if possible.

After doing these 23 steps, you will have things somewhat under control from having gone off sugar and some of your favorite foods and cleaners.

Check your pH every few days, to see if there is any difference in your pH level. Within a week try another test strip; your pH test should show between 6.5 and 7.5 in the healthy range. You will be greatly surprised if you do these steps every day and stick to them. This does not mean you're automatically healthy, but it does mean you're on your way to a healthier life. It is an indicator where your pH needs to be so your body can start to heal itself. This should give you hope and a good starting point. Try and make this a lifestyle by changing your eating habits. Hang in there and you can make a huge difference in your health and the way you feel. It does get easier, and it really does work.

Many people don't stop to think that they might be deficient in nutrients because they have no symptoms of disease. This can be far from the truth, so don't wait to get started on a superior nutritional supplement program. Let this book be your wake-up call. Carry it with you as a reminder, as I do. Dr. Joel Wallach, Ph.D., author of *Dead Doctors Don't Lie* says, "Every animal and every human being that dies of natural causes dies of nutritional deficiency diseases."

As I mentioned earlier, in 1999, after I had my prostate cancer operation, my doctor told me he had removed all the cancer, saying that "it looks good." A few days later my wife, who fortunately works in the medical field, saw something wrong in the paperwork regarding my operation. She went directly to the hospital lab and found out that my doctor had not removed all the cancer and had cut through some of the cancer cells in my body. The hospital lab told her I had "positive margins" which meant there were still cancer cells that had not been removed. From that day forward I became *obsessed* with researching everything I could find out about how to battle the cancer that was still in me, for if I didn't do something drastic, it was eventually going to come back to kill me.

TEN VERY IMPORTANT THINGS TO DO

Here's a list of things I did to start changing my diet for a healthier life, and to help get rid of my cancer. I found in my research that these topics help all diseases and not just cancer.

1. **Water:** We need plenty of pure fresh water for our bodies to work properly. Water is the "magic potion of life." Filtered spring water is what I drink; it seems to be the best water available for me.
2. **Detoxify:** Chemicals from food, pesticides, heavy metals, and byproducts from the environment build up in our bodies. We must detoxify our bodies to get these harmful substances out. Three excellent products for this purpose are; Natural Cellular Defense (zeolites), Modifilan, and Essiac Tea. There are many but these are three of the best.
3. **Diet:** This doesn't mean to lose weight unless you need to shed a few pounds, and if you're eating properly you will lose weight naturally. It does mean to drastically change your eating habits for the better and forever, by watching the kinds of food you do eat.
4. **Supplement:** Start using natural organic foods and nutritional products now. Get interested, get involved, and get prepared. If you have cancer, start reading about cancer diets and what you can eat. *www.cancertutor.com* is a good site to look at and a good place to start.
5. **Parasite Cleanse:** Your body and organs need to be cleansed of harmful parasites.
6. **Alkalize:** The pH in your body needs to be more alkaline than acid. When your body is too acidic you can start forming disease much more easily than when it is alkaline. See the Acid/Alkaline section in this book.
7. **Oxygenate:** We don't get nearly enough oxygen in our bodies. Breathe deeply often. Exhale by pushing as much of the old air out of your lungs as possible. Breathe deeply several times a day. Also, look into a good oxygen supplement at your health food store in a convenient liquid bottle form. You only need a few drops a day.
8. **Exercise:** Use it or lose it. It is extremely important that we keep fit and fight stress by exercising. Start with a short walk if needed and go from there. You will feel the difference when you're active and you get more oxygen into your blood and lungs.

9. **Sunshine:** We do need our sunshine! It is converted by our bodies into Vitamin D. Enjoy the sun, don't hide from it. Start slowly, about 15 minutes or less a day. Don't burn your skin and try not to use sunscreen if possible, it may cause skin problems or cancer. You can find good sun screen products at your health food store.

10. **Support:** Keep supporting your body by doing these 10 steps and don't give in by saying "It's not working" or "It's too expensive." Adjust your life to prevent health problems before they arise, and don't give up. Make it your new lifestyle and your new priority. This will be the support your body needs and you will see and feel the benefits as time goes by. But don't forget about your immediate family. They still need you and can give you a lot of support if you let them.

PRODUCTS I TAKE AND FIND VERY HELPFUL

The products in the following list are all excellent and are the ones I use. They are, in my opinion, some of the best on the market today. Remember, I had cancer, and it is now gone (from what my blood tests say) because I took the road less traveled to fight my disease with natural products. All of these products helped me win the battle with cancer, along with a positive attitude. These are the products I have taken and still take today. I am not advising **you** to take any of these products.

Some of the products in this book I mention by name brands and others by what they are used for. They are not in alphabetical order but close to the order in which I take them during the day. Look in the reference pages to find more great information on these products.

I have tried all of these in different combinations and I changed the rotation and amounts as time went by. Each of you can find your own products that seem to work the best for you. Now that my cancer is not showing a rise on my PSA blood tests, I will soon start to cut a few of these products from my diet to see if my PSA numbers stay in the safe range, continue to go down, or start to go up again within the next three months. But mostly, I will stick to the regimen that I have been on. (Several three-month blood tests have now come and gone with great results. My PSA numbers are still extremely low).

When a person's prostate has been removed during surgery, a PSA blood test is expected to be very low. The reason I return now to be checked is to continue to prove to myself that my cancer is still gone. Since I've had prostate cancer, having a PSA blood test every three to six months is an excellent way to check for a rising PSA level. This would indicate the reoccurrence of active cancer cells that my body is not killing.

All of the following products are very important to me. However, I will pick fourteen, out of this list, I think are the most important when cancer is present. They are: 1, 4, 5, 6, 7, 8, 11, 12, 18, 21, 23, 39, 40 and 41. For at least a year and a half I took everything on this list, most of them four times a day. This is where I would start again if needed. This is not counting good fresh water, number 26 on the list. As you know, water is a must, this goes without saying. Make sure you always drink the correct amount of water anytime, anywhere, or anyplace. Always try to drink filtered or bottled water that's easy to take along with you.

At this point, now that I can say my cancer is gone, I am consistently using nine of these products. They are 5, 10, 12, 14, 15, 17, 23, 40 and 41 and others when needed. As I keep learning I will add or maybe change some products.

Please make sure you have read the Exculpatory Note in the front of this book. Never take any new products if you're pregnant or nursing and never take or give anything in this book to infants or children without consulting an alternative doctor who knows about these products. Always keep these types of products far out of reach and out of sight of children. I am not suggesting you take these products at all. You have to make that decision for yourself about any products or medication you take. Remember, this book is for information only.

1. Essiac Tea: This is excellent for flushing the body of chemicals and toxins that have built up over a lifetime. You can purchase the herbs or the liquid. There are three different programs to follow plus a maintenance program. Ask an expert at your local health food store about these options. I started with one bottle at a time and followed the directions. Take 2 ounces every 12 hours on an empty stomach.

2. Flor-essence: Also an excellent chemical flush that is ready to drink. This has the same herbs as Essiac Tea plus a couple extra. Take 2 ounces, dilute with an equal amount of water, twice a day, one half hour before breakfast and one half hour before your evening meal.

3. Agrisept: Helpful for killing yeast, mold, herpes, candida, parasites, fungus, the onset of cancer, salmonella and so forth. Use as directed on the bottle.

4. Clarkia: Dr. Hulda Clark developed this product and has proved it will kill parasites. I took 12 to 15 drops in water three times a day, 30 minutes before meals, as directed on the bottle. You can also order these in capsule form from her website.

5. Paw Paw herb: This is one of the newest herbs on the market and works excellent for all types of cancers. I take one capsule, with food or without, four times a day as directed on the bottle.

6. The Budwig Diet: This is a mix of two or three tablespoons of flaxseed oil with highest lignan content and half a cup of 2% low-fat cottage cheese. Dr. Budwig developed this diet and says that the mixture of these two products will cure cancer. These need to be mixed together well before eating. Eat as a meal or snack and eat this every day.

7. Immutol: Excellent for boosting the immune system to help fight off cancer and disease. Follow the directions on the bottle.

8. Red raspberries: Ellagic acid comes from this berry and is said to kill cancer cells. I was taking two capsules four times a day.

9. L-glutathione: A great antioxidant. I followed the directions on the bottle.

10. *Lactobacillus reuteri:* A superior probiotic which is extremely important for better digestion, energy, and nutrition absorption, and inhibits the growth of harmful bacteria. Also look for Mega Flora (brand name) which is also excellent. Follow the directions on the bottle.

11. Vitalzym enzymes: Without enzymes, life would not exist. Follow directions on the bottle.

12. Modifilan: A brand name of the brown seaweed (fucoidan) known to kill cancer cells. It is a natural food. I take two to six capsules a day as directed on the bottle.

13. Multiminerals: I take one or two capsules or liquid every day, very important. When I'm taking one ounce of ProVitamin (#23 below) I only take one multimineral.

14. Vitamin B complex: I take an extra supplement every day, whether it's capsule or liquid.

15. Quercetin with bromelain and vitamin C: An important flavanoid needed in our diet. Follow the directions.

16. Super Omega complex with chromium: Oils and acids that our bodies need. Follow the directions.

17. Carlson's fish oils and shark liver oils are very good oils. I take two to four a day. Follow the directions.

18. B-17, also called leatrile: (Apricot seeds) is said to kill cancer cells. I have eaten 5 to 15 a day with no problems at all. Follow the directions.

19. Black Salve: Externally and/or internally: Helps to rid the body of cancer. I took this product internally and followed the directions.

20. Barlean's Greens: A "powdered greens formula" that will work wonders for improving overall health. I take two heaping teaspoons a day mixed in water.

21. Noni Juice: A wonder juice said by many to fight cancer. Follow the directions.

22. Barlean's flax oil with highest lignan: Excellent product for omega-3, 6, and 9. Follow directions on the bottle. If using the Budwig Diet you do not need to take more flaxseed oil.

23. Pro Vitamin Complete: This is a whole-food liquid supplement with all the nutrients you need in liquid form, vitamins, minerals, amino acids, trace minerals and more. I take One or two shot glasses a day. Follow the directions on the bottle.

24. Candex: A yeast management system which has natural enzymes to help control candida albicans.

25. PH strips: Needed to check alkalinity and acidity in the body. Follow the directions.

26. Water: The most important of all. Drink at least eight 8-ounce glasses a day of clean, fresh water with no additives. This means no water from a faucet.

27. Stevia: I use for a sweetener. Capsules, liquid, or powdered, at your health food store. Use as directed.

28. Teaga Tea: An herb that is said to help fight disease by helping the body to heal itself. Use as directed.

29. Kambucha Tea: Used for thousands of years or more as a health tea. Good for the whole body. I have used this off and on for years as I needed it. It works wonders.

30. CLA: An oil that helps fight cancer and other diseases. This product is also good for weight loss. Use as directed on bottle.

31. Glutathione (GSH): Helps to detoxify your body of poisons. Use as directed on bottle.

32. Lycopene: Helps to fight cancer. Use as directed on bottle.

33. Acai: A super fruit from the rain forest and a great antioxidant. Use as directed.

34. Okra-Pepsin-E3: Helps to clean the intestines so nutrients may be absorbed. Use as directed.

35. Maitake, reishi, and shitake mushrooms: Known to help fight cancer. I have taken two capsules twice a day. Follow the directions.

36. Fiber: Many of these products mentioned have fiber. Make sure you get enough.

37. Coral calcium and magnesium: Found in mineral supplements and foods. Helps fight cancer and disease and helps to keep the body alkaline. Used in the body for almost every function. Magnesium chloride is also excellent.

38. Olive oil, coconut, macadamia nut, grape seed, safflower and sesame oils. These are all good for you and are good for cooking and sautéing.

39. Pau d'Arco: An herb used widely in Africa for fighting cancer and disease. Use as directed.

40. Natural Cellular Defense (NCD): A product made from the zeolite family of minerals. This type of zeolite, sold as NCD, is a negatively charged volcanic mineral in a liquid solution that removes toxins and heavy metals from our bodies. This product does have a U.S. patent. The patent shows this product is a cancer killer and disease fighter. If you have cancer you *must* read this patent. Go to: *cancer.naturalcellulardefense.net*. This site also explains the great benefits of zeolites and how they work in the body.

41. Aerobic Oxygen: Extremely important in today's decreased oxygen environment. Oxygen empowers your immune system and sustains health and vitality. Inadequate oxygen in the body will decrease the effectiveness of the immune system and lead to oxygen deprivation (hypoxia). Aerobic oxygen is not a hydrogen peroxide product as some people think.

42. Remember to juice vegetables on a regular basis. Juicing good, raw, organic produce is like supercharging your body. It is excellent for your health and very tasty. You can use juice for a meal replacement. Try replacing one meal a day by juicing a large glass of vegetables. If you're weak from disease, or need help, have someone do this for you. If you're in a hurry, stop by a juice bar on your way to or from work or at lunch. While you're there, think about having a shot of wheat grass while waiting for your juice. Remember, you need your vegetables, lots of vegetables. Try to make sure they're organic.

These products do cost money, like everything else, and you're probably wondering how to fit them into your budget. If you're as desperate as I was, you'll want to do everything possible to find something that works for you. I started with one or two of these products, studied and learned more as I cut other foods out. This gave me more money to spend on the products I needed. I always have a good nutrition book with me to read and I'm constantly finding out more ways to fight disease and stay healthy.

Start looking around your health food store and farmer's markets for organic foods. Find organic foods with no sugar or artificial sweeteners that are ready to eat instead of candy, muffins, or bagels. Start driving by those fast-food restaurants and smile knowing your goal is better health. Get used to new products and foods and start eating more raw foods. Don't return to eating sugar and junk foods as you may have before. Give your body the chance it really needs to start healing itself.

The new foods you will discover may come from a health food store, but this doesn't mean to "grab it and eat it" because you're starving. Being hungry is not a bad thing, for most of us, unless you're malnourished. Take your time and look at the labels. Think about what you've been eating and remind yourself *why* you're changing your eating habits for the better. When you're hungry eat something healthy. Grab some raw vegetables or raw nuts, chew them up well and chase them with some fresh carrot juice or water.

The author says, "Cancer is a symptom of an ineffective immune system, it is not a death sentence. Give your body the right amount of water, the correct foods and herbs for healing and detoxifying, and nutritional supplements so it will work correctly and help boost your immune system to start the natural healing process. Your body is made to heal itself, I'm living proof that it really works.

WHY DO WE NEED PRODUCTS LIKE THESE?

Do we really need products like the ones listed? Of course we do, now more than ever. The environment we live in puts monumental stress on our lives. Some of this comes from polluted air, chemicals, and insecticides in and on our foods, vegetables, fruits, meats, milk, and the chlorinated water we drink. It comes from industrial smog from our factories, environmental pollution, pollution caused in the Chernobyl accident and others. Vehicle pollution and military and commercial jet planes polluting our air also take a huge toll on us daily. More and more of our food is now grown using genetic modifica-tions and chemicals. Our fast-paced lives push us to choose more fast foods and processed foods over fresh foods. Our careers, finances, and private lives add to the daily stress we live with, and our bodies become overloaded. These are some of the biggest reasons why we need every advantage to stay healthy.

In the westernized world we live in today, our U.S. medical schools are producing medical doctors with very little knowledge of nutrition or nutritional products. We have to take the responsibility for our own health, our family's health, and our grandchildren's health in the future. Just look at the path we have chosen to go down. Since many of our medical doctors cannot help us with the majority of our needs in the nutritional field, we need to be talking to the professionals in the field of nutrition such as herbalists, alternative doctors, naturopathic doctors, nutritionists, and so on.

As we move into the future with our health problems, let's hope the problems of curing disease diminish as the emphasis on better nutrition grows and becomes more of a priority. Many of us are starting to wonder what's going wrong, and why there's more and more disease now in younger and older people alike. With our unhealthy diets, disease is now becoming everyone's problem. Hopefully, preventing disease, starting from birth, will be in our near future as more and more parents and professionals realize these problems and start growing our foods without chemicals and pesticides.

On May 18, 2004 the U.S. Surgeon General, Richard Carmona, said it right. He said, "We must become a nation of prevention; we were too long a nation of treatment."

THE CANCER DIET I USE

By this time you're probably wondering what you can eat and what you can't, right? Take a look at my cancer diet below. Take another look at *briancalkins.comsimplevscomplexcarb.htm* and *www.cancertutor.com*.

If you want to reverse your cancer you *must* reverse and change your diet. This is a very big step for most people. Let me show you what I eat and show you the diet I used to helped get rid of my cancer. I am still eating this way today. I am now starting to expand my diet by eating a little more meat and fruits, working them back into my diet now that my cancer is gone. But now I only eat free-range meats, organic eggs, and organic fruit. I have lost 30 pounds, feel at least 20 years younger and have more energy than I can remember. This diet helped me win my fight with cancer with no ifs, ands, or buts about it. When I found out my cancer was returning again to kill me, I didn't have much of an appetite knowing I needed to drastically change my life and my diet again. The thing about this is, after my operation I still cheated a little on the sweets and carbs because I didn't know the impact these kinds of foods would have on my body. Even when I knew that my doctor had not removed all the cancer from my body, I had not educated myself enough to realize the impact of it all, to see the whole picture. I was relying on my doctor way too much, thinking everything would turn out OK some way, somehow while I was taking the meds he gave me. So I guess I needed an extra kick in the butt to get me going and make me realize I needed to get very serious again, even more than before because it might be my last chance. The best part of drastically changing my diet is that I still eat this way today and feel great. I don't cheat by eating sugar or junk foods, even at the best of parties, get-togethers, or holidays. *Just a little sugar can offset all the good you're doing while fighting your disease.* If you do find that you messed up, and ate something without thinking, don't beat yourself up. Just get back on the right track and move forward and don't look back. Always be positive in what you're doing and it will help fight your disease.

I try to eat an "80/20" diet, which means 80% raw vegetables and 20% cooked foods. When cooking your vegetables, cook them lightly steamed or lightly stir-fried with a little olive or coconut oil. Below are the foods I eat today. Purchase and read *A Cancer Battle Plan, Sourcebook* by Dave Frahm. This is an excellent book.

In the morning, or any time during the day, you can eat small amounts of Ezekiel 4:9 Sprouted Grain Bread and Ezekiel 4:9 Tortilla Shells, but I don't eat more than one piece a day. Go to: *foodforlife.com.* This bread is much easier on your system, especially if you're allergic to wheat. It is inspired by a verse in the Bible. This bread is live food, rather than processed food, and has no flour in the bread at all. It contains sprouted grain, which is the best way for wheat and grains to release their nutrients. The sprouted seeds are more easily absorbed because the gluten, found in the seed coating, is destroyed by the sprouting process of the seeds. This will take the place of regular bread and is great to eat with anything, especially eggs. It also makes a great sandwich. Be careful and watch what you make your sandwich with no processed mayonnaises, ketchups, or salad dressings. Make your own organic sauces and dressings, buy organic ingredients and use them very sparingly or don't use them at all.

Eggs are very nutritious, cooked or raw. Some people who are allergic to cooked eggs can eat them raw. People are concerned about eating raw eggs and contacting salmonella, but the risk is said to be very small. Make sure your eggs are fresh when you crack them open. Always eat organic eggs so you pass up the toxins. The egg carton will say "free range" or "organic." Eggs are good for us, despite what we grew up thinking. They are filled with nutrients and are very high in protein.

In the cancer diet I use, I do not use margarine or honey at all on Ezekiel bread or the tortilla shells. I use a light coating of butter, organic almond butter, or extra-virgin olive oil. Raw nuts such as almonds, walnuts, brazil, macadamia and pistachios are excellent, but no peanuts or peanut butter. Peanuts are said to have fungis and pesticides in them. Natural almond butter is good. Apricot seeds (from a health food store) taste better to eat with other nuts because they are bitter in taste. Pumpkin seeds and a high- quality greens formula containing spirulina and chlorella are also excellent. Buy a big container of a super "green food formula" in powdered form, like Barlean's Greens, and use it.

Eat all the vegetables you want. Try to start with at least 50% of your diet in raw vegetables, and work your way up to 80%. Watch the amount of carbs you are consuming very closely. It's extremely important to try and cut out all carbs, except vegetables, from your diet. Some vegetables are higher in carbs than others. One is corn which may also contain mold. Another vegetable, the (white) potato, is also very high in carbs. Remember, most carbs you eat are turned into sugar by your body. I sometimes have half of a sweet potato, which is much healthier. I also eat soups, organic and mostly vegetarian, with low or no salt. If salt is needed add a little sea salt, but no rice, pasta, or noodles. Very small amounts of meat are okay only if they are free range. Legumes and beans such as navy, pinto, kidney, black-eyed peas and others are high in carbs. They are good for us to eat and are high in vegetable protein but they are not a complete protein and are missing some of the eight essential amino acids. As my mother used to say, "Eat your beans with corn bread. It makes a complete protein."

Since cancer is present in my life, I seldom eat legumes because of the carbs, but legumes and beans are very healthy. What I do is look in the book called *Eat Right For Your Type*, that I mentioned earlier, to find out what type of beans agree with my body, and then I know for sure. When I do eat beans occasionally, I only eat small amounts. When fighting my cancer, I didn't eat legumes at all. Remember, since they are medium to high in carbs your body will use them as a form of sugar. So watch your intake of legumes while fighting cancer, sorry. Keep smiling and think positive. It does get easier.

Fresh fish is great to eat, if cooked well done to kill parasites, but I don't eat any canned fish or tuna. I try and eat only deep-water ocean fish that I know don't come from polluted lakes and waters, and not farmed fish, which are fed with toxic chemicals. These can be high in mercury and other toxins. Wild ocean fish may also have mercury and other toxins in them, but usually not as concentrated. Go to a health food store where they serve prepared food, and ask if they use free range meat or deep-water fish in their soups or other foods.

I eat small amounts of free-range chicken and turkey, just enough to mix in with a salad. Ask at the salad bar if they use organic vegetables and free-range meats. Salads with vegetables, nuts, and naturally nested (organic) eggs mixed in are great with a small amount of dressing like balsamic vinegar, olive oil, or flaxseed oil, added for taste. You can also eat spinach, sprouts, radishes, cucumbers, squash, tomatoes, red chili peppers, and all other types of vegetables unless they don't agree with you but, again, watch the potatoes and corn. Start adding more vegetables to your diet and start eating more of them raw and organic. The more raw organic vegetables you can eat, the better. But if you do cook them, only lightly steam or lightly stir-fry them.

Carrot and beet root juice mixed together is great. Add about 1/4 beet juice to 3/4 carrot juice. You can add celery, wheat grass and/or other vegetables as well. It makes a good mix that tastes great and is very healthy.

Add a little ice and blend it in, it's better cold. I find it best to drink this in the morning, on an empty stomach, along with taking my supplements, but anytime during the day is great and two or three times a day is better. Another often overlooked tip is to make sure your ice is not from your water supply if you're using city water, because of the chlorine, fluoride, and sometimes other toxins found in city water. Vegetables are excellent for the body. Another excellent vegetable we sometimes overlook is asparagus. It is amazing what this plant will do for the body. A small book to read on this one is called, *Asparagus Can Do It For You* by Theodore A. Baroody D.C., N.D., Ph.D. You'll be amazed!

I try not to eat any dairy products at all. This diet means no yogurt, milk, ice cream, sour cream, whipped creams and so forth, except when following the "Budwig Diet" for cancer I talked about earlier. With this diet you can use organic 2% low-fat cottage cheese and flaxseed oil with highest lignan content available. It will say this on the bottle. This diet is a great cancer fighter and will help fill you up. Mix them together well in a bowl before eating, or a blender can be used. I found I didn't need a blender to accomplish this.

Once in a while, I will now eat a small slice of hard cheese for a treat, but only once in a while and only Tillamook cheese. Tillamook and a very few other companies that make dairy products and cheese don't use the genetically engineered growth hormone rBGH, which is said to cause cancer. If needed, go back and read the article on milk or check your computer search engine for "Tillamook cheese rejects the use of rBGH." When you have time, call or send Tillamook a letter and let them know they have your support in this effort. Their address is: Tillamook Cheese Co. 4175 Highway 101 North, Tillamook, OR 97141. Phone 503-815-1300. Go to this website to read one of the papers to pressure Tillamook into using the bovine growth hormone in the products. *www.organicconsumers.org/monsanto/cheese022105.cfm.*

I don't use iodized table salt and I use very little black pepper, which can be acid forming in the body. Pure sea salt is good in small amounts, and cayenne pepper is excellent. Remember I had cancer. I did not drink alcohol while fighting my cancer. I now have a half glass of red wine once or twice a week. I never use tobacco products at all. I do not drink coffee, which also means no decaf. Decaf means the caffeine has been taken out, usually by some type of toxic chemical process. Coffee is also very acidic. Some blood types have an easier time with coffee than others. If your blood type is okay with drinking coffee, think about using the Gano coffee I mentioned in this book. Herbal teas with no caffeine are great. Also, organic dandelion detox tea, red clover tea, and green teas are excellent cancer fighters. Use stevia as a sweetener if needed. It's a sweet herb found at your health food store.

People with cancer should eat very little fruit until their cancer is gone, except for fruits that can help kill cancer cells. One of these fruits is the purple grape. Make sure you eat it all, the seeds, the skin, and be sure to crunch the seeds up with your teeth. The seeds are where all the cancer-fighting nutrients are, so crunch them up. It is always best to buy organic, but if you can't find organic make sure you wash the grapes and other fruits extremely well. They have high amounts of spray (pesticides, insecticides, and other chemical toxins) on them, which are poison. These toxic chemical sprays used on fruit may cause cancer, so wash them well. See the section on NCD (zeolite). This is a super detoxifier and a great cancer fighter.

If your fruit is not organic, wash each individual piece with warm organic soap and water or put them in a bowl or sink with a 50-50 solution of apple cider vinegar and water for 15 minutes to wash off the chemicals. Or, use some type of natural fruit chemical remover especially made for fruits and vegetables, and rinse them extra well. You should be able to find a natural product to remove chemicals from fruit at your health food store. Also, wash organic fruits well before eating.

Red raspberries and pomegranates are excellent. They have a large amount of ellagic acid, especially in the seeds. Strawberries, pineapple, and apricots are also great fruits for fighting cancer. Bilberries, cranberries, and black currants are low in sugar and provide high amounts of vitamin C, fiber, folic acid and phytochemicals. If you're going to eat fruit, eat it separately from your vegetables and meat during a different time of day, and eat them in small amounts, even the ones good for fighting cancer. Different types of food need longer to digest, using more enzymes. Some foods ferment, when eaten together, causing gas and stomach cramps especially when you're eating raw fruits with cooked meats. It is best to eat them separately unless they are all cooked together.

Also, blueberries are not to be forgotten. They are very low in sugar and are super high in antioxidants. In addition to fighting cancer and heart disease, blueberries help to fight your body's aging process.

Fruits have natural sugars and one that you might know about is fructose, a natural form of sugar that can feed cancer like other refined sugars. Although it is nothing like refined sugars, research shows the fructose in fruit can still be used as fuel by cancer cells. Don't get me wrong, according to *www.mercola.com* and many other websites fruit is excellent for us but people with cancer should watch their intake of all sugars until their cancer is gone. Remember, cancer loves sugar.

Use your imagination about what to eat after reading this cancer website. *www.cancertutor.com*. If you're serious about changing the way you eat, then stick to a diet that will help fight your disease. Make sure you read the labels on the back of everything you buy and remember no sugars, artificial sweeteners, carbs, processed foods or flour at all to start with. Before you put it in your mouth, think.

Special diets are essential for life, and you're fooling yourself if you think you can get away without eating "live foods" that contain nutrients and enzymes instead of "dead foods" that don't contain any real nutrients. Now that you have read about my cancer diet you may want to go a step further in great nutrition for your particular blood type. I would recommend that you take a look at this great book. It's called, *Cancer, Fight It with the Blood Type Diet* by Dr. Peter J. D'Adamo. I have mentioned this book before, but I need to mention it again.

Again, *always* drink lots and lots of pure fresh water. Water that comes from your tap, even if it's chlorine and fluoride free, is still running through your pipes. *Filter it.* If needed, go back in this book and read about water. Watch your pH level; you should be *alkaline*. Supplement with oxygen. Cancer *cannot* live in an oxygen environment.

If you're eating the wrong kinds of foods (carbs, sugars, artificial sweeteners, junk foods, processed foods, etc.), smoking, or drinking excessively while using nutritional products, supplements, herbs, or a cancer diet to fight your cancer, stop before it's too late. You can cancel out, or severely alter, any natural treatment plan you might be on. Eating the wrong foods will offset the results, wasting money and valuable time fighting your cancer.

Additionally, when you go out to eat, be sure not to cheat on your diet plan and always ask to be sure there are no added sugars or chemicals such as MSG or other added chemicals on, or in, your food. Waiters are used to being asked such things these days with more people eating more naturally and with organic foods. Watch out for the coatings and sauces as well. Again, be aware of everything you put in your mouth.

Stay away from heavy oils unless you are sure they are healthy oils. Be very careful about what you put in your mouth and the types of oils the food is cooked in. As I mentioned before, I only use olive, coconut, grape seed, safflower, sesame or macadamia nut oils to cook with and a few others I take for their nutritional benefits. These are flaxseed oil, borage oil, a good quality fish oil (Carlson Norwegian Salmon Oil) and shark liver oil. Or I sometimes only take a Super Omega Complex, a mixture of all these healthy oils except shark liver oil. Shark liver oil contains the most concentrated amounts of alkylglycerols. This can also be found in mother's milk and bone marrow. It is high in vitamin A and D and is also high in Omega 3. Alkylglycerols help to speed up healing and help the fight with cancer.

New studies have shown that a high intake of ALA from flaxseed oil, which contains omega-3 fatty acids, is associated with an increased risk of prostate cancer. Dr. Udo Erasmus, Ph.D., says the way fats and oils affect the prostate has led some conclusions to be inconsistent. He states that, "Several research labs have found ALA is one of the most powerful growth stimulants for human prostate cancer cells in tissue culture." But then, another study in this same website below shows, in 1985, GLA and ALA killed prostate cancer cells and did not affect normal cells. Take a look at this website below and see what you think about this very touchy subject. I have used the Budwig Diet, which uses flaxseed oil, for a couple of years and my PSA numbers went down. Flaxseed oil did not make my PSA numbers go up. But then I must also say, when I started with flaxseed oil my prostate had already been removed. Go to: *www.rightfatdiet.com/articles/udo/flax_prostate_expanded.htm*. Also read the book, *Fats That Heal Fats That Kill*, by Udo Erasmus.

What I do now is buy just the flax seeds and grind them up in a coffee grinder and sprinkle them over the food I eat. Or you can also buy gelatin capsules from your health food store and fill them up with your ground-up flax seeds to take them along with your other supplements. It is also said, high levels of selenium, up to 200 micrograms a day, cuts prostate cancer risks in half.

When you're eating foods that are cooked, let this list be a quick reminder. Eat small amounts more often if needed. You can eat larger amounts of vegetables but try not to stuff yourself. Start eating smaller amounts and be smarter about what you're eating.

Choose foods like:	Avoid foods like:
Baked	Breaded
Broiled	Creamed
Grilled	Fried or deep fried
Poached	Basted with heavy sauces
Roasted	Au gratin
Steamed	Alfredo
Sautéed	Ala King
Stir-fried	Light or heavily burned
Butter (sparingly)	Margarine

It's hard to know what kind of snacks to eat when disease is present. Below are snack foods I eat that are very healthy and very low in natural sugar. I only started to eat these after my PSA numbers from my blood tests went way down.

Below are a few foods that are very low in natural sugars that I still eat today. I would not recommend eating these products until you get a handle on your cancer. But, if you must, eat them in small amounts. After the product name below I will say which of these products I ate more of than the others when fighting my cancer.

1. Spirulina Ginseng Balls. This is one I ate while fighting my cancer and is a very healthy snack made from spirulina greens that I mentioned earlier. When I found that my PSA numbers were going way down, I tried these spirulina balls and I still eat them today. I started by eating one a day, mainly because they contain only a very small amount of natural sugar, which I was doing my best to stay away from. I now find myself eating more

of these than any other snack. Spirulina is a superb food. Every order from this company is made fresh when they receive your order. You might want to go back and read about spirulina, and then check these out at: *www.john@bettylousinc.com* or call 1-800-242-5205.

2. Greens Plus+ Energy Bar. I ate these bars about once a week, for a treat, while fighting my cancer. This excellent-tasting energy bar is full of organically grown greens, quinoa sprout powder and non-GEF soy protein high-energy herbs, and has no added sugar except a very small amount in the form of honey. It has no salt, corn syrup, hydrogenated oil, synthetic sweeteners, preservatives, or GEF. It is also alkaline to the body when eaten and cold processed, which keeps in all important nutrients. It comes in two flavors, natural and chocolate, and both are wonderful. Check out their website at: *www.greensplus.com.*

3. Boomi Bars. I ate these snack bars occasionally while fighting my cancer and now I eat them often. There are several different kinds of Boomi Bars. Some are lower in natural sugars than others. They have homemade natural ingredients and are vegetarian and gluten free. If purchasing, stay with the ones lowest in sugar like Healthy Hazel, Cashew Almond, or Perfect Pumpkin. They're all excellent. Go to: *www.boomibar.com* or call 1-800-440-6476.

4. Check out the "Pro Bar" at your health food store, if they carry it. A recreational or sports store, like REI, may also carry it. While fighting my cancer I ate no more than half of a bar once a week just to have something different and filling. The Pro Bar contains 17 whole foods, has a broad spectrum of nutrition, and is 70% raw food. This one is higher in carbs and natural sugars but you only need a small amount to take your hunger away. If you have cancer, eat only a quarter of this bar every couple of days, or stay away from it until you get your cancer under control.

5. Goji Berries are an excellent snack. I ate only a handful of these every couple of days and not at the same time that I ate

half the Pro Bar or other dried fruit. The Gogi berry is a super healthy dried fruit that supplies the body with immune system polysaccharides and other nutrients and tastes a little like raisins. These dried berries are pinkish red in color and can be found at your local health food store, or go to your computer's search engine.

6. Raw nuts are great and very healthy. After reading the book *Cancer, Fight It With The Blood Type Diet* by Dr. Peter J. D'Adamo, I ate only nuts that are good for my blood type when fighting my cancer. Be sure you're not allergic to nuts before eating any. I like pumpkin seeds, almonds, and walnuts, which are good for my blood type. Also, when eating apricot seeds (pits), you can mix them with almonds and/or other nuts. Apricot seeds are fairly bitter to eat.

7. Juicing or eating raw vegetables are the very best for snacking or for a meal. Wheat grass, sprouts, carrots, beets, cabbage, broccoli and many other vegetables will definitely help fight your disease. It will also make an extremely healthy snack. I always try to juice vegetables or eat them raw every day. Find a blender that leaves the fiber in the juice and always do your best to eat organic.

8. Dried fruits are always a great snack. Find out what fruits are good to eat for your blood type, instead of wondering and worrying. Most dried fruits are high in natural sugar or have sugar added to them. Be careful when eating dried fruits. Remember, cancer loves sugar. I did not eat any dried fruits, except small amounts of Wolf Berries, until my PSA numbers were dropping considerably.

9. Chocolate? Yes, you can! Chocolate is not a bad thing *if* it's the right kind. It's what the chocolate has in it that makes it bad for the body. Organic dark chocolate is the only kind I will eat and only if it's a least 85% pure organic dark chocolate with a very low amount of natural sugar. Make sure you check both the percentage of dark chocolate and the amount of natural sugar before you purchase that yummy reward for being good after eating your vegetables. This is not something you want

to eat right away when fighting cancer. Wait until you have no cravings for sugar. This kind of chocolate is not found at your local candy shop although some grocery stores are starting to carry different varieties. A health food store is where to go. And again, remember, cancer loves sugar. If you have cancer, be extremely careful. I didn't eat any chocolate at all until I knew my cancer was on its way out and then I ate only one small little piece. I don't really consider this type of chocolate, candy. Check out Dagoba Organic Chocolates. One kind of Dagoba chocolate is called "Eclipse 87% Extra Dark" and is very low in sugar. Find it at your health food store or log on to: *www.dagobachocolate.com.*

10. If your body is saying "I need something crunchy," try Mary's Gone Crackers.These are crispy crackers with a great taste. They are wheat free, gluten free, with no added oils or fats and no hydrogenated or trans-fatty acids (bad oils). They can be found in four different flavors; organic rice, quinoa, flax seed, and sesame seed. Add a little organic cheese and you've got it made. They're also great to eat by themselves. Check it out at *www.marysgonecrackers.com.*

11. TERRA exotic vegetable chips have a crunch like potato chips but are made from root vegetables like sweet potatoes, parsnip, batata, taro, yucca. These chips are tasty, have no trans-fat, and are good for you. Check them out at *www.terrachips.com.*

Before you eat anything, always be sure you know exactly what you're eating in every single bite. And then go for it and eat organic, raw, and whole foods. Try to eat 80% raw vegetables and 20% cooked foods. Work your way up to this amount. Your stomach will thank you. Ease your way up to eating more raw foods, and you will see a much healthier you soon after.

<u>NOTES</u>

NOTES

PART 18

WAKE UP, BEFORE IT'S TOO LATE!

WHAT ARE WE TO DO?

You might ask yourself what you can do about all this. If you're a family person with children, or maybe you have a loved one with problems of failing health, you need to have a plan.

One thing you could do is call your senator and congressman to express your feelings and concerns. Let them know what you think about the junk foods in our schools our kids are eating. I personally know. I work at a high school with up to 2,000 students. Also, ask them about genetically engineered foods, the rise in obesity, diabetes, and the rise in heart disease and cancer which have been around even longer, and are now getting worse. Then ask about all the different types of toxins that are in everything we eat and drink unless you grow it or buy organic foods. If they seem unconcerned, something is wrong.

Other things you could do are move to the wilderness, dig your own well, grow your own food in your organic garden, free of sprays, bug and weed killers; raise your own cows, goats, and chickens without putting chemicals or hormones in their feed. Or, you could start thinking of better and smarter ways for you and your family to live in the city and be healthier by eating the right kinds of foods and drinking the right kinds and correct amounts of liquids.

You need to start changing your eating habits now. Start by drinking spring or filtered water instead of pop, sugar waters, sweetened juices, or artificially sweetened beverages. Buy fresh vegetables, organic if you can find them. Go to your neighborhood market and ask if the vegetables are organic or if they were sprayed or grown using weed killers, bug killers or any other chemicals or insecticides of any kind. Stop eating junk foods, processed foods, and fried foods cooked in the wrong kind of oils with trans-fatty acids. Canned vegetables are not the best choice over fresh vegetables. Quite often they have been overcooked and overprocessed, causing them to have very few nutrients. Many canned foods also contain way too much salt. Frozen vegetables are much healthier and if packaged correctly, hold nutrients longer. Buy only organic meats, eggs, and poultry that are free of chemicals and hormones. Read where it says "organic" or "free range" on the carton or ask at the store. Otherwise, don't buy them. The chemical additives and sprays in and on the food we make, and the animals we eat, are passed on to you and your children.

So, I say there is hope for a total cure for cancer and not just a way to put cancer in remission, but real hope. I don't believe we will ever see a world completely free of cancer with all the pollutants and chemicals around us. But, I do believe with all the great products on the market and organic foods, we do have a real chance. However, we must be ready and willing to drastically change our lifestyle and eating habits for the better. This doesn't have to be done all at once but the faster the better.

The first step should be a simple test strip to check your body's pH. Learn how to keep your body in an alkaline, and not acidic, state by what you eat and the nutritional supplements you take, or should be taking. Then, get started on a super whole-food nutritional supplement your body desperately needs. Remember, your body is screaming for nutrients.

You also need to cleanse your small intestines so your body can absorb all the nutrients you put into it. Consult with a homeopathic doctor when starting to do any kind of cleansing or detoxifying of your body unless you already know what to do. Start eating more vegetables and fruits. Drink lots of pure, but not distilled, water, and wean yourself off processed sugars and foods. I recently tried a mango in season and WOW, now I buy them by the flat, usually nine at a time. Just by taking these few first steps you will start to rebuild your body and jump-start your immune system for a great new healthier lifestyle. Within a few weeks, you'll feel those nasty little aches and pains start to disappear; then you will know something good is starting to happen.

The road a person chooses to take when it comes to cancer treatment is very personal, and says a lot about what the person's belief is about treatment. It also shows what they know, and don't know, when it comes to believing what their doctor has to say and what their natural fears may be. It is said that these are the reasons why most people line up for conventional cancer treatment, trusting in our medical system, and hoping that it won't fail them. Be very aggressive with how you treat your disease! If you do nothing, it could cost you your life!

Look into the websites and books I've mentioned in the reference pages as a study guide. Get professional advice right away from your medical doctor, naturopathic doctor, or alternative doctor. Study the references I've mentioned. The correct nutritional products are extremely important and have made a very big difference in my life. Otherwise, I would not have taken the time to write this book. Please remember, before embarking on such a life-changing path, many medical doctors know very little about what I have written in this book and/or do not believe in natural healing.

All written material listed within this book, aside from direct quotes, is from what I have learned. The story I have told is my personal battle fighting and conquering cancer. There is a lot of great information here, and a wealth of information listed in the reference pages. So please, take your time while reading through this book.

It's time to wake up folks, the sooner the better! Too many people think the time to start with nutritional supplements is when they find out they have a disease. But the real time to start is now, before you contract one. It is called *prevention*, so make it a priority in your life and your body will thank you for it. Start now.

Believe it or not, we're all made out of the same thing. If it costs you a little extra to get started on the road to health, you're worth it. Try skipping one night a week out for dinner with your family and fix something healthy at home. If you really start to eat healthier, a little bit at a time, you won't notice such a big difference in your wallet or pocketbook when purchasing nutritional products when you finally decide to completely switch from processed foods to a more healthy diet. You'll find out as you get healthier, your aches and pains will start to disappear, you'll have more energy and feel like going out for a walk because you're not so tired, drugged out, or have that run-down feeling. And, hopefully, someday you will also say, "Cancer and disease don't scare me anymore."

SAVE OUR SUPPLEMENTS NOW
BEFORE IT'S TOO LATE!

Leaders in Washington D.C. are working right now, in 2005-06, to restrict our access to the vitamins and dietary supplements we depend on for our health, happiness, and a better life. Some of the Central American Free Trade Agreement (CAFTA), which comes under the World Trade Organization (WTO), may be restricting or even banning dietary supplements in the United States very soon as they already have in Australia and some European countries.

The Dietary Supplement Health and Education Act (DSHEA) of 1994, a law that preserves our right to safe, natural nutritional supplements, passed Congress only because of 2.5 million letters congressmen received from people like you and me who know how important nutritional products are in our country today. Despite the outpouring of support people showed for nutritional freedom in our country, a handful of senators continue working hard to bring about "adverse event reporting" (AER), which will rip away our freedom of personal choice in taking vitamins and supplements. In a time of skyrocketing insurance and health care costs, this could be a national tragedy. When our elected officials in our government want to take away our right to choose what vitamins and supplements we want and don't want so we can stay healthy, it is a very direct way of showing what really is happening in our government. What will it be next?

The Codex Alimentarius Commission, organized in the 1960s by the United Nations, is responsible for consolidating food supplement policies between all nations in the world. Codex Alimentarius, translated from Latin, means "food code." Under this policy, even the basic vitamins and minerals we buy would require a doctor's prescription. The new European Union has adopted this new policy and it went into effect in 2005. Other countries are said to follow suit very soon by passing new laws in favor of these new policies and regulations. The United States signed up to Codex, thus binding all of us to these ridiculous regulations. It is said, if we don't act on this together, as a nation, we will very soon be going to our medical doctors to receive nutritional vitamins and supplements by prescription only. Today, some of the congressmen we trust are slipping these types of laws as riders onto larger bills to get them passed without our knowledge.

Become a voice for supplement choice now, before it's too late. Scientists have proven thousands of plants do have excellent healing abilities, not only for disease but for pain management and depression. These plants were placed here on this planet for us to use to heal ourselves from disease, pain, and suffering. I believe, as many others do, these products do not need to be regulated by our government as our prescription medicines are.

Log on to *www.saveoursupplements.org* and *www.citizens.org* and find out what you can do to help. This could turn into a very scary situation, especially when *you* need, or want, these supplements that have been taken off the store shelves and are now regulated by our government. Go into these sites. Send a letter, already prepared, to your senators and congressmen in Washington D.C. It's easy and it works.

Also go to *stopfdacensorship.org* so we, people of our nation, can have a better look at what information the FDA is keeping from us. Once again the people of America have to defend themselves in telling our elected officials at home and in Congress to leave our supplements and our rights to choose alone. I might not be here today if I hadn't had that right to choose about my cancer.

Ask at your health food store if they have free copies of *Energy Times*. On page 16, Volume 16, No.1 of the January 2006 issue of this health magazine, it has an article about this, and names two senators as key figures in AER legislation. You can also subscribe free to *Energy Times* at 1-800-937-0500. Australia recently had about 1,200 vitamins and supplements removed from their store shelves shortly after Australia signed up to CAFTA, as the United States did in June or July 2005.

Thomas Jefferson once said, "The doctor of the future will give no medicine, but will interest his patients in the care of the human frame, in diet, and in the cause and prevention of disease." There's that word *prevention* again.

Now that you have read this book, let me ask you this. Are you being medicated until the day you die because of some type of disease? I was headed down that same road but I turned around and ran the other way. That road, to me, was dark and gloomy and was definitely not the road for me. I saw my opportunity and jumped all over it. I'm not saying that I won't ever take prescription medications again because I don't know what might happen and where life will take me. As mentioned earlier, I do believe in my medical doctor but I don't believe there is a miracle drug for everything. As I moved ahead with fighting my cancer, I notice I was having better results with natural products than with prescription medication. So, as time went on, I went with what my body responded to the best and here I am today.

This book is the result of my obsession with saving my life. It's not easy to change the road we travel and all the bad habits we picked up along the way. But if you want to stay healthy during your life, you definitely need to make a change for the better, or you may not be here tomorrow. Think of it this way. If you have cancer, the information in this book will only help you. What do you have to lose? Life is too short to throw all your eggs in one basket. I ask you to keep an open mind and also look for new products and research that is constantly coming into view for us to stumble upon if we're so lucky. I realize that it takes time to step out of our comfort zone, but be aware of what is out there and move forward and learn.

If my cancer was ever to reappear, the very first thing I would do is read this book again and study all the great websites and books available in the reference pages. Remember, it took me years to read through hundreds of websites and other great information to come up with what you are reading right now. I believe miracles really do happen. I wish you all the luck and great health, whatever road you choose to travel.

NOTES

<u>NOTES</u>

Reference Pages

Here you will find books, brochures websites and other forms of information that I use and find very helpful and effective in fighting disease. There is a wealth of information here. There may be words listed in these pages you're not used to seeing or using every day. Use the glossary in this book, or use *www.wikipedia.org* for word definitions.

WEBSITES

These websites are in alphabetical order by the products listed on the right. Some of these websites may have been deleted or outdated. New websites may have replaced the old. If a site you go into is not working try your computer's search engine.

www.	Product and information
naturalhealthschool.com/acid-alkaline.html	Acid-alkaline balance
collagendiet.com/grapefruit_seed_extract.htm	Agrisept-l
lovetohelpyou.com/body.html	Agrisept-l
shirleys-wellness-café.com/alert.htm	Alert to comsumers
alkazone.com	Alkaline booster
PeopleAgainstCancer.com	Alternative cancer therapy
alternative-doctor.com/cancer/kelly.htm	Alternative cancer ways
whale.to/m/quotes6.html	Alternative doc.
hps-online.com/fastcolbacwin1.htm	Antibiotics and acidophilus
betterhealthcenter.com	Antioxidants
mdschoice.com/text/topical/antioxidants.htm	Antioxidants
Qray.com 1-888-616-1180	(Arm band) pain relief
barleans.com/literature/index.html	Articles
mnwelldir.org/docs/cancer1/altthrpy.htm	Aspartame
doorway.com	Aspartame and other info
herbs-oils.tripod.com/aspartame.html	Aspartame danger
mercola.com/forms/sweet_misery.htm	Aspartame danger
risingsunhealth.com	Black Salve
smarthealthcenter.com/cancer.html	Black Salve/cancer
frequencyrising.com/bodycleanses.htm	Body cleanses
barleans.com/products/books.html	Books

blpublications.com/html/	Books
newstarget.com	Books
cancer.org/choiceoftherepy.htm	Books
huldaclark.com	Books and herbal remedies
naturalcures.com	Books and more
rainforesttools.com	Book / CD/Acai
udoerasmus.com/fatsmain.htm	Book/flaxseedoil/ prostate cancer
preventcancer.com/avoidable	Breast cancer book
flaxoflife.com	Budwig Diet
seekingcenter.com/healing/03_personal/ budwig/diet.html	Budwig Diet recipe
hill.ccsf.cc.ca.us/~jinouy01/drbudwig-diet2.html	Budwig Diet, & info
cancure.org/budwig_diet.htm	Budwig Diet for cancer
mysite.wanadoo_members.co.uk/ cancermagic/index.html	B17 laetrile & more
cancersalves.com	Cancer
krysalis.net/cancer.htm	Cancer
http:/home.bluegrass.net/~jclark/cancer_buster.htm	Cancer
cancer.gov/newscenter/1971-nca	Cancer Act of 1971/Nixon
cancertutor.com	Cancer and other info
whale.to/w/politic.html	Cancer article
cassandabooks.com	Cancer Books
cancer.org/choiceoftherepy.htm	Cancer books & tapes
home.bluegrass.net/'carrie73/doctors_clinics.htm	Cancer clinics
alternative-cancer.net/Mexican_hospitals.htm	Cancer clinics in Mexico
texascancerclinic.com	Cancer clinic in Texas
stopcancer.com	Cancer, diets, brain, DMSO
www.beating-cancer-gently.com	Cancer Free (book)
herbsforcancer.com/cancer.html	Cancer herbs
cancure.org/choiceoftherapy.htm	Cancer info
cancertutor.com/other/nocancer.html	Cancer info
healingdaily.com/conditions/ cancer-prevention-measures.htm	Cancer info
racingsmarter.com/process_sugars.htm	Cancer info
doctormurray.com	Cancer info
cancertutor.com	Cancer info, diets
mnwelldir.org/docs/nutrition/sugar.htm	Cancer loves sugar
cancer-coverup.com/story/story/-a.html	Cancer politics
alkalizeforhealth.net/loxygen2.htm	Cancer prevention

w3.bluegrass.net/~jclark/small_intestine.htm	Cancer products
alternativecancer.us	Cancer products and info
home.bluegrass.net/'carrie73/protocol_911.htm	Cancer protocol 911
ncra-usa.org/pdfs/resources/nca_overview.pdf	Cancer, reenergizing the war
aicr.org.uk	Cancer Q&A's
pureessencelabs.com	Candex
mercola.com/2002/aug/14/con_ola1.htm	Canola oil
alternativecancer.us/antioxidant.htm	Cantron
carctolusa.com/	Carctol, herbal cancer
	supplement
mercola.com/forms/carlsons.htm	Carlson's Fish Oils
sandmountainherbs.com	Catalog of herbs
heartfoods.com	12 day flush
essence-of-life.com	Cesium chloride products
drcranton.com/chelation/allgood.htm	Chelation
drcraton.com/chelation/find.htm	Chelation: area find
evenbetternow.com/environmental-toicity.htm	Chemical/metal toxicity
com/chlorellacomposition.htm	Chlorella
newstarget.com/zoo8527.html	Chlorella, defense/cancer
chlorellafactor.com/chlorella-spirulina-04.html	Chlorella / spirulina
iternethealthlibrary.com/environmental-health/	Chlorine/cancer/
chlorine-and-cancer.htm	heart disease/ageing
cancer.org	Cigarette smoking
drclarkia.com	Clarkia for parasites
shop.toolsforhealing.htm/	Clarkia (tincture)
cosmonet.com/rife/drhuldaclark	Cleanse herbs
mercola.com/2004/nov/13/clorine_water_cola.htm	Clorine, tap water, diet cola
discount-vitamins-herbs.net/	CLA benefits
bestmall.com/wp/tonalin	CLA oil
mercola.com/forms/coconut_oil.htm	Coconut oil
phoffoods.html	Coffee and ph
ganobrandcoffee.com/greg	Coffee, Gano brand
krchealth.com/colloidal_story.htm	Colloidal silver
healthycolon.net/	Colon cleanser
allnaturalinfo.com/herbal_cleanse.htm	Colon & parasite cleanse
proimagenutrition.com	complete vit/min
optimal.org/peter/easycron.htm	CRON diet
detoxify.com	Detox 1-800-338-6948
joi.ito.com/archives/2002/10/26/	Diet Coke
is_diet_coke_bad_for_you.html	

mercola.com?2002/may/8/distilled-_water.htm	Distilled or natural water
mercola.com/article/water/distilled_water.htm	Distilled water
dmso.org	DMSO
proevity.com	Docs and glycos/phytos
whale.to/cancer/quotes.html	Doctors quotes
mercola.com/article/cancer/cancer_options.htm	Dr. Moss questions chimo
notmilk.com/thekillers.html	Drugs / bacteria
eatright.htm	Eat right for your blood type
mercola.com/2005/jul/23/water_toxins.htm	Environmental toxins
coastherbal.com/	Enzogenol, Slim Sweet
srherbs.com	Enzymes, digestion
sweetvibranthealth.com	Essential sugars
healthproductsusa.net/7essiacinfo_health.htm	Essiac tea
essiac-info.org	Essiac Tea
rense.com/general53/ms.htm	Excitotoxins, MS
haciendapub.com/article27.html	Excitotoxins
foodforlife.com	Ezekiel 4:9
	Sprouted Grain Bread
fact55.com	F.A.C.M. Alter. Med.
fda.gov/opacom/backgrounders/msg.html	FDA position on
fda.gov/bbs/toxins/answers/ans0072.html	FDA position on
florahealth.com	Flor-Essence (detox)wholly-
water.com/fluoride.htm	Fluoride in our water
waronaids.com/foods-that-kill.asp	Food additives
godsdirectcontact.com/vegetarian/alkalineoracid.html	Food chart acid/alkaline
udoerasmus.com/articles/udo/flax_prostate.htm#n-3	Flaxseed Oil/cancer
rightfatdiet.com/articles/	Flaxseed Oil/cancer
udo/flax_prostate_expanded.htm	
acaiforlife.comfaqs/acai_benefits.cfm	FrutaVita Acai fruit
fungi.com	Fungus
safecoffee.com	Gano healthy coffee
netlink.de/gen/Fagan.html	GE foods
organicconsumers.org	Genetically altered foods
GEfoodalert.org	Genetically altered foods
blilliston@iatp.org	Genetically altered foods
alaskawellness.com/mar-apr04/antioxidant.htm	Glutathione
whey2health.com/glutathione_antioxidant.htm	Glutathione
immunotec.com/glutathione/page.asp	Glutathione
glyconutrients-facts.com	Glyco- and phytonutrients
glycoscience.com	Glyconutrients info

glycoinformation.com	Glyconutrients info
goji-berry-juice.net	Goji berry juice
sevenstories.com/	Got Milk book
nutribiotic.com	Grapefruit extract
briancalkins.com/	Great info
theanswertocancer.com	Great cancer book
jennyleenaturals.com	Greens
barleans.com	Greens
living fuel.com	Greens / Thera Sweet
hacres.com	Hallelujah Acres Diet
inmotionmagazine.com/geff4.html	Hazards of GEF and crops
energytimes.com	Health magazine
cancerplants.com	Herbs
cancersalves.com	Herbs
nativeremedies.com	Herbs
cancerchecklist.com/cancerherbs/cancerherbs.html	Herbs
herbs for cancer.com	Herbs
www.cancer.org	History of cancer
superbherbs.com	Hyloronic acid/arthritis
holographichealth.com	In-Sync, pain relief
altcancer.com/ioncleanse.htm	Ion foot cleanse machine
mercola.com/2003/may/24/cancer_contagious.htm	Is cancer contagious
kalisessentials.com/ingredience/klarkia	Klarkia for parasites
cajunernie.com	Kombucha mushroom tea
kombuchatea.co.uk/index.asp	Kombucha Tea
heartfoods.com	Lecithin and flush
w3.bluegrass.net/~jclark/print_dosage.htm	Laetrile/Vit.B17
sciencedaily.com	
mushroomscience.com	Medical mushrooms
altered-states.net/healing/cancer.htm	Medical ozone and cancer
aspartameispoison.com	Micheal Fox story
	(also see books)
salvemgoldmandds.com/detox2.htm	Mercury detox
metabolictypingdiet.com/index2	Metabolic dieting
mercola.com	Metabolic test, trans-fats
mercola.com/forms/mt_test.htm	Metabolic type test
jrussellshealth.com/microwaves.html	Micro-waving
rense.com/general7/gotmilk.htm	Milk
freedom-you.com/	Milk, baby food etc.
mercola.com/2000/july/30/milk.htm	Milk & cancer breast/

	prostate
preventcancer.com/press/books/got.htm	Milk dangers
my.athenet.net-mkd/minerals.htm	Minerals
trccorp.com	Minerals
mushrooms.com	Mushroom health info
nuconceptsinc.com/fungus.htm	Mold info
natural-health-solutions.net	Oxygen
pure-noni-juice.us/noni_comparison.htm	Noni comparison
nonialoha.com	Noni Hawiian
sharenoni.com/science.htm	Noni juice
wellnesshour.net/mambo	Nutritional talk show
lcompnutrition.com/sea-vegg.html	Ocean blends of kelp
naturesaide.com	Oral chelation
organic consumers.org/sos.cfm	Organic Consumers Association
thefutureisorganic.net/organicnutri.htm	Organic is healthier
oxygenhealingtherapies.com/ my_ozone_doctor.com.htm	Ozone clinics
cancure.org/choiceoftherapy.htm	Ozone clinics and therapies
drstallone.com	Ozone clinic in Arizona
lightparty.com/health/medicalozone.html	Ozone therapy
cancertutor.com/cancer/ozone.html	Ozone therapy
lightparty.com	Ozone therapy and more
oxygenhealingtherapies.com	Ozone therapy/cancer
behealthyamerica.com	Ozone therapy/cancer
urezone.com/clark	Parasites and more
jointpainremedy.com	Natural pain relief
eazol.com	Natural pain relief
alternativecancer.us/pawpaw.htm	Paw Paw herb
pawpaw.tv	Paw Paw herb
healthysunshine.com/paw-paw-cell-reg.htm	Paw Paw order
naturessunshine.com	Products/Paw Paw order
naturestools.com	Paw Paw report
mercola.com/2003/aug/20/peanuts_health.htm	Peanuts
peopleagainstcancer.com	Personalized cancer info
maverickranch.com/	Pesticides in our beef
digestinol.com/paradox.shtml	Polysaccharide molecule
ph-ion.com	pH test and books
essence-of-life.com/info/phpaper.htm	pH paper, info
focus-on-nutrition.com	pH paper, shark liver oil

redflagweekly.com/storm_warings/poison.htm	Poison for profit
renewlife.com	Probiotics
americanlongevity.net	Products / Vital'e
pcaw.com/newsite/events/pcaw	Prostate cancer info
moduprost.com	Prostate health
calcompnytrition.com/proxenol.html	Proxacine and Proxenol
wellnessletter.com/html/ds/ds/dsQuercetin.php	Quercetin flavonoid
askjeeves.com	Questions and answers
monsanto.com/protivadr.greene.com/2t_1680.html	rBGH
foxbghsuit.com/bgh4.htm	rBGH hormone in milk
caers@cfsan.fda.gov	Report an adverse drug
caoh.org/vision-vitamins.html	Reseasonable products
deodorant-stones.php	Safe deodorant
saccharides.net	Sales
living-foods.com	Salt
pinsight.com/~gssi	Sea salt
spirulina.html	Spirulina
mercola.com/2000/dec/3/sucralose_dangers.htm#	Splenda
mercola.com/fegi/pf/2004/jul/21/splenda.htm	Splenda
holisticmed.com/books/bkfood.html#stevia	Stevia
mercola.com/article/sugar/sugar_cancer.htm	Sugar
mercola.com/fegi/pf/2000/oct/8/sugar_cancer.htm	Sugar and cancer
mercola.com/2005/may/4/sugar-_dangerous.htm	Sugar dangers
mercola.com/forms/livingfuel.htm	Super greens
naturalproductsinsider.com/ hotnews/492315146.html	Supplements, save billions
saveoursupplements.org	Supplements under attack
cancenewswithview.com/hnv/hot_new_vidiosl.htm	Sweet Misery (video)
livingfuel.com	Thera Sweet
psa-rising.com/eatingwell/turmeric.htm	Termeric herb
alternativecancer.us/pawpaw.htm	Test kit, compare chart
globallight.net	Tiaga tea
rense.com/general137/toth.htm	Toothpaste
gifam.org/npcleaning.htm	Toxins
bodypurenow.com	Toxin removal pads
mercola.com/2001/july/21/trans_fat.htm	Trans-fat
essiacinfo.org	True story of healing cancer
ralphmoss.com/ukrain.html	Ukrain and cancer
ukrain-drug.net/web/webspreed/index.html	Ukrain
pancreas-ukrain.comeffectukraincancer.htm	Ukrain

liverenewedlife.com/us_senate_document264.htm	U.S. Senate Doc., #264
drwong.info	Vitalzym enzymes
worldnutrition.info	Vitalzym inf.
tuberose.com/water.html	Water
colonhealth.net/free_reports/h2oarticle.htm	Water
levaquell.com	Water is life
macrobiotic.org/thalass.htm	Weak cancer patient diet
mercola.com/forms/whey_healthier.htm	Whey drinks that are good
firstshake.com	Whey/Dream protein
collagendiet.com (Agisept-L)	Weight loss, parasites, Candida, yeast
123healthguide.com/products/bath-&-body-	Xylitol, sorbitol, sannitol
en.wikipedia.org/wiki/Xylitol	
mercola.com/2005/feb/19/common_toxins.htm	10 most common toxins

My personal websites I use for products are listed here:

www.	Product	Phone when not using websites
proimageteam.com/25005	Pro Vitamin Complete	1-800-323-3681 ID# 25005
mywaiora.com/691120	Natural Cellular Defense	1-866-699-2467 ID# 691120
mynsp.com/superherbs	Paw Paw, Immune Boost, and more	1-800-223-8225 ID# 17952996
ganobrandcoffee.com/greg	Low acidic coffee no sugar chocolate with Ganoderma mushroom added to coffee. Website orders only	

For more info and products go to www.defeatcancer.org

Health Newspapers, Pamphlets, Articles, and Magazines

AARP: The Magazine, Jan/ Feb., 2005 "A Dire Warning," Dr. J. Wallach

Alaska Wellness Magazine, March-April Edition 2004

"Dietary Supplements Under Imminent Threat," Vitamin Research News, Nov., 2004

Energy Times, July/August 2005, free subscription 1-800-937-0500

"Gano Coffee" (The Healthy Coffee) 1-800-373-6076

Health Science Institute, July 2003 "Nature's Perfect Food"

Health Perspectives "Practical Insights into the World of Natural Healing, An Important Message to Women: Lignans Reduce Risk and Spread of Breast Cancer"

Health Perspectives "Practical Insights into the World of Natural Healing, Omega-3 Oils Prevent Heart Attacks," Jade Beutler, R.R.T., R.C.P

"Journal Of The Science Of Food and Agriculture" 2003; 93 (14)

Men's Journal, July 2003, "The Fruit That Packs a Punch" Tyler Graham

People Against Cancer, "The Alternative Therapy Program for Cancer" P.O. Box 10, Otho, Iowa 50569, 1-515-972-4444.

"Prevention," by Media Vision 2005, L.C., Vol.1, number 1 1-800-368-3038

"Sunshine Sharing," Vol. 14 No.7 (Regarding Paw Paw herb) 818-994-6693

"Trans-Fat: What Exactly Is It, and Why Is It So Dangerous" Dr. Mercola

"Ukrain": For info on healing cancer contact: Anne Beattie 1-718-636-4433

Vitalzym, Total System Support (pamphlet) 1-877-626-3130

Wall Street Journal, The; April 18, 2003, "Acaci Replaces Wheatgrass"

Washington Post, The; Aug., 11, 2004: Page F

Water,"The Snowbird Diet," Donald S. Robertson, M.D.

"Wellness Report," Vol 40 No. 1, (Paw Paw herb, 1-888-225-6601) James South, M.A., modified by Dr. Richard Newman

Books, Movies, Tapes, and CD's
Alphabetical by Title, Tape, or CD

Title	Author
A Cancer Battle Plan Sourcebook, A	Dave Frahm
Alkalize or Die	Dr. Theodore A. Baroody
Alive and Well	Dr. Binzel
A New Health Era	William H. Hay
Ask the Doctor, Nature's Liver Remedy: Milk Thistle Extract	Dr. Michael T. Murray
Aspartame Disease, an Ignored Epidemic	H. J. Roberts, M.D.
Beyond The 120-Year Diet	Roy Walford M.D
Bypassing Bypass Surgery	Elmer M. Cranto M.D.
Breast Cancer Prevention Program, The	D. Steinman, S. Levert, S. Epstein
Breuss Cancer Cure, The	Rudolf Breuss "A Cure Therapy"
Cancer Cover-Up, The Neal Deoul Story	Dr. Neal Deoul
Cancer, Cure and Cover Up	Ron Gdanski
Cancer Doesn't Scare Me Anymore	Dr. Day
Cancer Free	Bill Henderson
Cancer Industry, The	Ralph W. Moss
CLA, Conjugated Linoleic Acid	Lane Williams 1-888-779-7177
Colostrum: Nature's Gift to the Immune System	Beth M. Ley 1-888-367-3432
Cover-Up, the Neal Deoul Story	Neal Deoul (A Must Read)
Cure for All Cancers, The	Hulda R. Clark, PhD, N.D.
"Dead Doctors Don't Lie" (Audio Tape)	Joel Wallach B.S., D.V.M., N.D.
Diet and Supplement Plan For Cancer	Robert O. Young
Eat Right Four (4) Your Type	Dr. Peter D' Adamo
Fats That Heal Fats That Kill	Udo Erasmus
Flood your body with Oxygen	Ed McCabe
Genetically Engineered Foods, A Self Defense Guide for Consumers	Ronnie Cummings and Ben Lilliston
Genetically Engineered Foods, Science On The Edge	Karen E, Bledsoe

Get With The Program	Bob Green; Oprah's personal trainer
Global Light Network	Tiaga Tea, Order 888-236-210
Glutathione, Master Antioxidant: *The Next Vitamin C*	Russell Manuel M.D.
Got (Genetically Engineered) Milk	Samuel Epstein
Guide to Nontoxic Treatment and Prevention	Ralph Moss PhD
Healthy Fats For Life: Preventing and Treating *Common Health Problems With Essential* *Fatty Acids*	Lorna R. Vanderhaeghe
Herb Finder, Total Cleanse	Loren N. Biser, 1992 801-575-6247
Herbs for cancer, History and controversy	Ralph W. Moss, PhD
How Cancer Politics Have Kept You in the Dark	Dr. Diamond and Dr. Cowden M.D.
How to Fight Cancer and Win	William L. Fischer
Incurable Diseases	Dr. Richard Schulze
Killers Within	Michael Schnayerson and M. Plotk
Left For Dead	Dick Quinn 800-229-3663
Let's Eat Right To Keep Fit	Adelle Davis
Medical Ozone and Cancer	Ed McCabe
Metabolic Typing Diet	William Wolcott and Trish Faher
Milk A to Z	Robert Cohen
Milk: The Deadly Poison	Robert Cohen
Nature's Medicine Chest (Book & CD)	Dr. J. Klein, PhD 866-541-7919
Naturopathic Physician	Vital Communications, 1997
NONI, How Much, How Often: *Nature's Gift To Cancer Patients*	Isa Navarre 1-800-748-2996
Noni: Nature's Amazing Healer	Dr. Neil Solomon
Noni Revolution, The	Rita Elkin, M.H.
One Answer To Cancer	Dr. William D. Kelly D.D.S., M.S.
Pain Free In Six Weeks	Sherry A. Rogers, MD

Politics And Healing	Dan Haley
Politics Of Cancer Revised, The	S. Epstein and J.Conye
Prostate Health In 90 Days	Larry Clapp
Restoring Your Digestive Health	Jordan Rubin, PhD
Safe Shoppers Bible	Samuel Epstien and David Steinman
Seeds Of Deception (movie)	Order: 1-800-955-0116
Sick and Tired, Reclaim Your Inner Terrain	Robert O. Young
Slim Sweet	Martha M. Christy
Splenda: Is It Safe Or Not?	Dr. Janet Hull
Stopping Cancer At The Sourse	M. Sara Rosenthal, PhD
Sugar Blues	William Duffy
Sugars That Heal	Emil Mondoa, MD
Super Size Me (movie)	movie rental store
Sweet Misery	(movie) Order: 1-800-955-0116
Sweet Poison	Dr. Janet Hull
Total Health Program, The	Dr.Joseph Mercola
Trust Me I'm A Doctor	Dr. J. Wallach
Ultimate Cancer Conspiracy, The; Vitamin B17 and Laetrile	JoeVialls
Ultimate Weight Solution, The	Dr. Phil
What The Bleep Do We Know!?	(Movie) www.whatthebleep.com
Whole Soy Story, The	Dr. Kaayla Daniel
Who's Afraid Of A Cure For Cancer, The Struggle For An Alternative Cancer Drug	Elmore Thun-Hohenstein
World With Out Cancer	G. Edward Griffin 877-479-3466
Your Body's Many Cries For Water	F. Batmanghelidj, MD

List Of Authorities

Abbott, Isabeela, Dr.
Adomo, D., Dr.
Albrech, William, Dr.
Bailer, John, Dr.
Balch, James, M.D.
Baroody, Theodore A., Dr.
Becker, Robert O., Dr.
Blaylock, Russell, Dr.
Brusch, Charles, Dr.
Budwig, Johanna, Dr.
Caisse, Rena
Carlson, Dr.
Carmona, Richard
Carrizo, M.D.
Clark Hulda, R., Dr.
Clifton, Leaf Dr.
Cowden, Lee, M.D.
D' Adamo, Peter, Dr.
Daniel, Kaayla, Dr.
Denao, Esteban, Dr.
Diamond, John, M.D.
Epstein, Samuel, Dr.
Erasmus, Udo, Dr.
Frahm, David
Guyton, Arthur C., Dr.
Harman, Dr.
Hay, William H., Dr.
Heinicke, Ralph, Dr.
Hill, John, D.C.
Hertel, Haus, Dr.
Hull, Janet, Dr.
Kafman, David
Koop, Everett, Dr.
Krebs, Ernest T., Dr.

Krebs, Dr.
Lee, Lita, Dr.
Lehmann, Soren, Dr.
Manuel, Russell
Marille, Nancy
McLaughlin, Jerry, Dr.
Mercola, Dr.
Mindell, Earl, Dr.
Mondoa, Emil, M.D.
Murray, Michael T., N.D.
Nordstrom, Bjorn, Dr.
Nieper, Hans, Dr.
Nowicky, Wassyl, J., Dr.
Olney, John, Dr.
Oster, Kurt A., Dr.
Pasteur, Louis
Pauling, Linus, PhD
Porter, Dr.
Price, Joseph, Dr.
Reign, Carl, Dr.
Schechter, Steven, Dr.
Skinner, Michael, Dr.
Wallach, Joel, PhD
Warburg, Otto, Dr.
Wilson, Pete
Way, Spencer, Dr.
Whitaker, Julian, M.D.
White, Milton, M.D.
Williams, Michael, Dr.
Wilson, J. Walter, Dr.
Wiseman, Richard, Dr.
Xing Nianzeng, Dr.
Zimen, Irwin, M.D.

Glossary

Below you will find some of the words that are not already defined in this book. If you need a better definition than you see here, or I have not included one that interests you, please go on line to *www.wikipedia.org* or *www.yahoo.com.*

Adjuvant: A pharmacological agent added to a drug to increase or aid its effect.

Aerobic Oxygen: Stabilized electrolytes of oxygen in a molecular form.

Alfa-Linoleic: ALA. A green food such as Barley greens high in unsaturated fatty acids containing many nutrients and Omega-3.

Alkaline: Also, Alkali which is the opposite of Acid or Acidic. The alkaline side of the pH range in the body.

Alkylglycerols: Gycerols derived from shark liver oil.

Annonaceous Acetogenins: New technology reproducing cancer-fighting analogs believed to halt the growth of cancerous tumors in humans.

Anthocyanins: A water-soluble pigment that reflects the red to blue range of the visible spectrum in plants.

Antioxidants: Chemicals that halt the oxidation of the nutrients (free radicals) they fight.

Anvirzel: An herbal extract which is nontoxic and is new in the fight with cancer.

Apoptosis: The destruction of cancer cells (cell death) due to activation by the digestive enzymes contained in the cells themselves.

Arginine: One of the twenty most common Amino Acids.

Artemisinin: A drug to test multi-drug-resistant strains of Falciparum Malaria.

Bastille: Prison or stronghold.

Benign: Any medical condition left untreated that will not become life threatening. Some benign tumors may be life threatening if not removed.

Bromelain: A collection of sulfur-containing enzymes.

Cachexia: Loss of weight, muscle wasting, fatigue, weakness, and unwanted anorexia seen with many cancer patients, usually close to death.

Carotenoid: A natural pigment in plants.

Chlorocarbons: Refers to hydrocarbons in which hydrogen atoms are replaced by chlorine atoms.

Chlorella: Single-celled algae and a Greek word meaning "small".

Choline: An essential nutrient. Not to be confused with chlorine.

Cis-isomers: Isomers are molecules with the same chemical formula. *Cis* means, "on the same side."

Cortisol: A corticosteroid hormone involved with the response to stress. It increases blood pressure and blood sugar levels, and suppresses the immune system.

DNA: (Deoxyribonucleic Acid) is a nucleic acid that specifies the biological development of all cellular forms of life.

Detoxing: Also called, detoxifying and detoxification is the removal of toxic substances from the body and one of the functions of the liver and kidneys.

Diketopiperazine: A class of cyclic organic compounds that result from peptide bonds between two amino acids.

Efficacy: The power or capacity to produce a desired effect.

Emu Oil: Oil of a flightless Australian bird.

Emphysema: A chronic lung disease usually from exposure to toxic chemicals and tobacco.

Endorphins: These are peptides (endogenous opioid biochemical compounds) produced by the pituitary gland. They have the ability to produce analgenia and a sense of well-being and may work in the body as natural pain killers.

Epidermoid: Benign tumor composed of cells that embryologically give rise to the skin and its appendages.

Fibrinolytic: A process where a fibrin clot of coagulation is broken down by the *Plasmin* enzyme.

Fibromyalgia: A debilitating chronic syndrome with pain and fatigue with a wide range of symptoms.

Flavonoid: A type of antioxidant or bioflavonoid.

Free Radicals: Also called radicals. Many forms of cancer are said to be the result of reactions between radicals and DNA resulting in mutation that affect the cell cycle leading to malignancy and disease.

Glucoronic Acid: The uronic acid of glucose the conjugates various substances in the liver so as to detoxify or inactivate them.

Goitrogens: Food plant species including cabbage, broccoli, cauliflower, rutabaga etc.

Histoplasmosis: An infectious disease caused by the inhalation of spores of hisstoplasma capsulatum. A influenza-like illness.

Hydroxcyl Radicals: Produced during the reaction of hydrogen peroxide.

Hypoxia: Less than adequate oxygenation of tissues and cells.

Inositol: A cyclic polyalcohol and a secondary messenger in a cell. Also inositol is a member of the B complex vitamins.

Laric Acid: The main fatty acid in coconut oil and palm kernel oil with a very low toxicity.

Lectins: Proteins of nonimmune origin that interact with sugar molecules. Lectins play an important role in the immune system.

Leptin: A protein hormone that plays a key role in regulating energy intake expenditure.

Lignan: Phytoestrogen antioxidant nutrient found in plants. Not to be confused with Lignin.

Linolenic: A polyunsaturated acid and an omega-6 fatty acid.

Linolenic Acid: Also called alpha Linolenic. An18 carbon polyunsaturated fatty acid with three double bonds. It is also an omega-3 fatty acid.

L-proline: One of 20 Proteinogenic units which are the building blocks of proteins.

Lycopene: Red carotenoid pigment. Photochemical found in tomatoes.

Lymphasarcoma: Sarcoma is a cancer of the connective or supportive tissue, (bone, cartilage, fat, muscle and blood vessels).

Mannitol: A sugar alcohol which is acidic. An osmotic diuretic agent and sugar substitute.

Minerals: Natural compounds formed through geological processes.

Neurotoxic: exposure to manmade toxins which alters the normal activity of the nervous system.

Neutrophils: A class of white blood cells, which are part of the immune system.

N-Nitroso: A functioning group in organic chemistry. Nitroso compounds.

Nitrosodientholamine: A well-known carcinogen.

Organic compounds: Molecules containing carbon with exception of carbides, carbonates, and carbon oxides. Many of these are protein, fats, and carbs.

Phosphatidyl: A phospolipid compound derived from soy lectins.

Phospholipid: A class of 4 lipids and a major component of all biological membranes.

Phytates: Phytic acid known as inositol henaphosphate or phytate in salt form.

Phyto-chemicals: A phyto-nutrient (antioxidants) compound found in plants.

Polyaromatic Hydrocarbons: Larger systems of benzene rings fused together are known. The molecular structure of which incorporates one or more sets of six carbon atoms connected by delocalized electrons.

Polyphenols: A plant chemical substance responsible for the coloring of some plants.

Polysaccharides: Relatively complex carbohydrates. Polymers made of monosaccharides and joined by glycosidic linkages.

Probiotics: A dietary supplement with beneficial bacteria which assist the body with natural occurring flora in the digestive tract.

Proteolytc enzyme: Aids in the metabolism of food-derived proteins in the digestive tract.

PSA: Prostate-specific antigen which is a substance that can be detected in the blood of men, which helps to determine if there may be prostate cancer.

Radical Prostatectomy: Complete surgical removal of the prostate.

Sarcoidosis: Immune system disorder (small inflammatory nodules) mostly in the lungs, but any organ can be affected.

Scrophularia: Also called Figwort. A herbaceous flowering plant.

Sorbitol: See Mannitol or Xylitol.

Spirulina: Blue-green algae with 13 species.

Superoxide Dismutase: An enzyme which changes the dismutation of superoxide into oxygen and hydrogen peroxide.

Systemic: Affecting the whole body.

Substantia Nigra: A layer of large pigmented nerve cells in the Messencephalon that produce dopainine. This can be associated with Parkinson's disease.

T-cells: A subset of lymphocytes that play a large role in the immune system. *T* stands for thymus, where the final stage of development occurs.

Taxol: Also called pacltaxel. A drug used in the treatment of cancer from the Pacific yew tree.

Tricalcium Phosphate: Bone ash which is one of the main combustion products of bone.

Villi: Also called villus, are tiny finger-like structures that protrude from the wall of the intestines for absorption of nutrients.

Xylitol: A wood sugar used as a sugar substitute.

Zeolites: A volcanic mineral. 48 types are known. One type is marketed as Natural Cellular Defense, in a liquid form, to be taken to fight cancer and other disease. This product has a U.S. Patent that shows certain types of cancer it kills.

Index

Printed in the United States
147884LV00001B/2/P

9 781933 973029